Contents

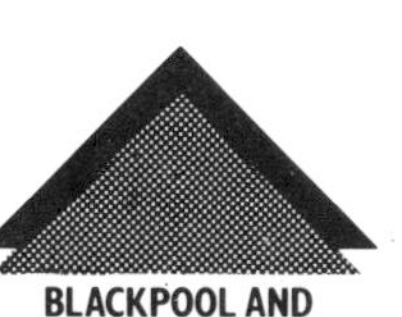

of Medicine

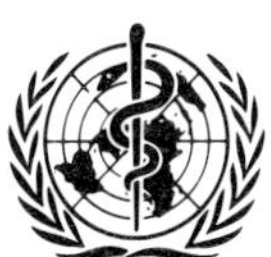

World Health Organization
Geneva
1993

WHO Library Cataloguing in Publication Data

Beaglehole, R
Basic epidemiology / R. Beaglehole, R. Bonita & T. Kjellström
1.Epidemiology I.Bonita, R. II.Kjellström, T. III.Title

ISBN 92 4 154446 5 (NLM Classification: WA 105)

Reprinted 1994 (twice), 1996, 1997, 1998 (twice)

TYPESET IN INDIA
PRINTED IN ENGLAND

91/9100—94/9924—94/10125—96/10830—97/11362—98/11908—28500
98/12117—Arrowhead—2000

Preface

Basic epidemiology has been prepared with a view to strengthening education, training and research in the field of public health. The need for this text became apparent during discussions between WHO staff and medical educators in many countries. Furthermore, responses to a questionnaire sent to members of the WHO Global Environmental Epidemiology Network (GEENET) demonstrated a strong desire for a WHO text on basic epidemiology.

The authors gratefully acknowledge the help received from a large number of colleagues. The first draft text was reviewed by an editorial group which included: Dr José Calheiros, Oporto, Portugal; Dr Vikas K. Desai, Surat, India; Dr Osafu Ogbeide, Benin City, Nigeria; and Dr Robin Philipp, Bristol, England. Valuable comments were also received from Dr Peter Baxter, Cambridge, England; Ms Jo Broad, Auckland, New Zealand; Dr Ruth Etzel, Atlanta, USA; Dr Charles du Florey, Dundee, Scotland; Dr Ichiro Kawachi, Wellington, New Zealand; Dr John Last, Ottawa, Canada; Dr Anthony McMichael, Adelaide, Australia; Dr Markku Nurminen, Helsinki, Finland; Dr Annette Robertson, Suva, Fiji; Dr Linda Rosenstock, Seattle, USA; Ms Judi Strid, Auckland, New Zealand; and staff in the WHO Division of Epidemiological Surveillance and Health Situation and Trend Assessment, the WHO Division of Development of Human Resources for Health, and the WHO regional offices. Ms Martha Anker, of the WHO Division of Epidemiological Surveillance and Health Situation and Trend Assessment, provided a major contribution to Chapter 4.

A pre-publication version was widely circulated in 1990; it was formally evaluated by 12 teachers of epidemiology and their students in 10 countries. The present version takes into account all the comments received during that review.

Production of this training material was supported by the International Programme on Chemical Safety (a joint programme of the United Nations Environment Programme, the International Labour Organisation, and the World Health Organization), the Swedish International Development Authority (SIDA) and the Swedish Agency for Research Cooperation with Developing Countries (SAREC).

Introduction

The essential role of epidemiology in the Global Strategy for Health For All was recognized in a World Health Assembly resolution in May 1988, urging Member States to make greater use of epidemiological data, concepts and methods in the preparation, updating, monitoring and evaluation of their work in this field, and encouraging training in modern epidemiology of relevance to the evaluation of approaches used in different countries.

This text provides an introduction to the basic principles and methods of epidemiology. It is intended for a wide audience, including professionals in the health and environment field involved in in-service training courses, undergraduate medical students, students in the other health professions, and other students needing an understanding of this field. The terminology used in this book is largely based on *A dictionary of epidemiology* (Last, 1988).

The purpose of this book is to:

- explain the principles of disease causation with particular emphasis on modifiable environmental factors;
- encourage the application of epidemiology to the prevention of disease and the promotion of health, including environmental and occupational health;
- prepare members of the health-related professions for the increasing need for health services to address all aspects of the health of populations, and to ensure that health resources are used to the best possible effect;
- encourage good clinical practice by introducing the concepts of clinical epidemiology;
- stimulate a continuing interest in epidemiology.

At the end of the course the student should be able to demonstrate knowledge of:

- the nature and uses of epidemiology;
- the epidemiological approach to defining and measuring the occurrence of health-related states in populations;
- the strengths and limitations of epidemiological study designs;
- the epidemiological approach to causation;
- the contribution of epidemiology to the prevention of disease, the promotion of health and the development of health policy;

- the contribution of epidemiology to good clinical practice;
- the role of epidemiology in evaluating the effectiveness and efficiency of health care.

In addition the student will be expected to have gained a variety of skills, including an ability to:

- describe the common causes of death, disease and disability in her or his community;
- outline appropriate study designs to answer specific questions concerning disease causation, natural history, prognosis, prevention, and the evaluation of therapy and other interventions to control disease;
- critically evaluate the literature.

A teacher's guide accompanies the present text. Obtainable from the Division of Environmental Health, World Health Organization, 1211 Geneva 27, Switzerland, it provides information to assist in the organization and delivery of the course, together with illustrations suitable for overhead projection, suggestions for examinations, and guidance on how the text can be used, evaluated, and adapted to the local situation.

Chapter 1
What is epidemiology?

The historical context

Origins

Epidemiology has its origins in the idea, first expressed over 2000 years ago by Hippocrates and others, that environmental factors can influence the occurrence of disease. However, it was not until the nineteenth century that the distribution of disease in specific human population groups was measured to any great extent. This work marked not only the formal beginnings of epidemiology but also some of its most spectacular achievements; for example, the finding by John Snow that the risk of cholera in London was related, among other things, to the drinking of water supplied by a particular company. Snow's epidemiological studies were one aspect of a wide-ranging series of investigations that involved an examination of physical, chemical, biological, sociological and political processes (Cameron & Jones, 1983).

Snow located the home of each person who died from cholera in London during 1848–49 and 1853–54, and noted an apparent association between the source of drinking-water and the deaths. He prepared a statistical comparison of cholera deaths in districts with different water supplies (Table 1.1), and thereby showed that both the number of deaths and, more importantly, the mortality rate were high among people supplied by the Southwark company. On the basis of his meticulous research, Snow constructed a theory about the communication of infectious diseases in general and suggested that cholera was spread by contaminated water. He was thus able to encourage improvements in the water supply long before the discovery of the organism responsible for cholera; his research had a direct impact on public policy.

Snow's work reminds us that public health measures, such as the improvement of water supplies and sanitation, have made enormous contributions to the

Table 1.1. Deaths from cholera in districts of London supplied by two water companies, 8 July to 26 August 1854

Water supply company	Population 1851	No. of deaths from cholera	Cholera death rate per 1000 population
Southwark	167 654	844	5.0
Lambeth	19 133	18	0.9

Source: Snow, 1855.

health of populations, and that in many cases since 1850 epidemiological studies have indicated the appropriate measures to take.

The epidemiological approach of comparing rates of disease in subgroups of the human population became increasingly used in the late nineteenth and early twentieth centuries. The main applications were to communicable diseases (see Chapter 7). This method proved to be a powerful tool for showing associations between environmental conditions or agents and specific diseases.

Modern epidemiology

The more recent development of epidemiology can be illustrated by the work of Doll, Hill and others who studied the relationship between cigarette smoking and lung cancer in the 1950s. This work, which was preceded by clinical observations linking smoking to lung cancer, expanded epidemiological interest to chronic diseases. A long-term follow-up of British doctors indicated a strong association between smoking habits and the development of lung cancer (Fig. 1.1).

Fig. 1.1. Death rates from lung cancer (per 1000) by number of cigarettes smoked, British doctors, 1951–1961

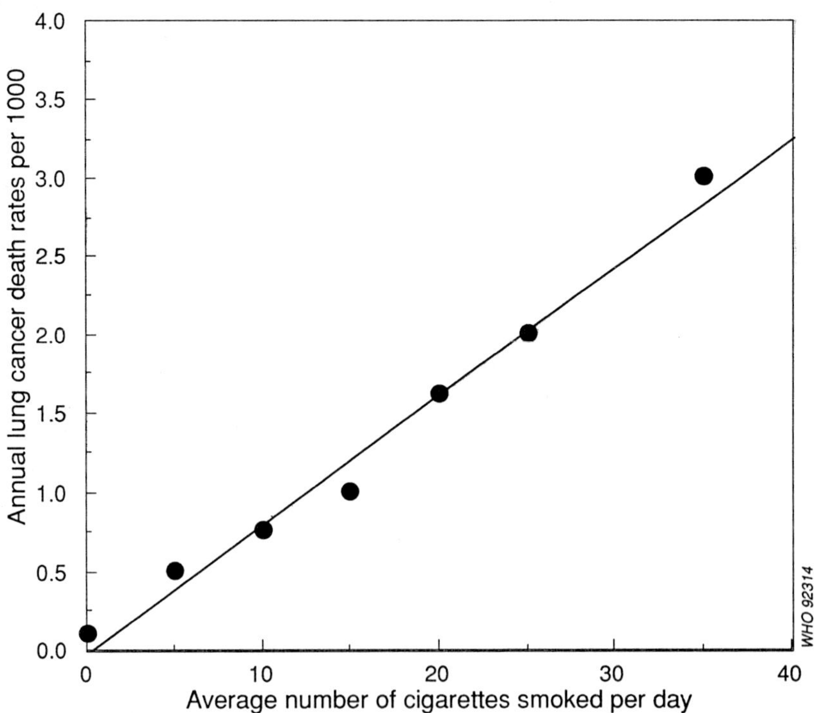

Source: Doll & Hill, 1964. Reproduced by kind permission of the publisher.

It soon became clear that, for many diseases, a number of factors contributed to causation. Some factors were essential for the development of a disease and some just increased the risk of developing it. New epidemiological methods were required to analyse these relationships.

Today, communicable disease epidemiology remains of vital importance in developing countries where malaria, schistosomiasis, leprosy, poliomyelitis and other diseases remain common. This branch of epidemiology has again become important in developed countries with the emergence of new communicable diseases such as Legionnaires' disease and the acquired immunodeficiency syndrome (AIDS).

Definition and scope of epidemiology

Epidemiology has been defined as "the study of the distribution and determinants of health-related states or events in specified populations, and the application of this study to control of health problems" (Last, 1988). This emphasizes that epidemiologists are concerned not only with death, illness and disability, but also with more positive health states and with the means to improve health.

The target of a study in epidemiology is a human population. A population can be defined in geographical or other terms; for example, a specific group of hospital patients or factory workers could be the unit of study. The most common population used in epidemiology is that in a given area or country at a given time. This forms the base for defining subgroups with respect to sex, age group, ethnicity, and so on. The structures of populations vary between geographical areas and time periods. Epidemiological analysis has to take such variation into account.

In the broad field of public health, epidemiology is used in a number of ways (Fig. 1.2). Early studies in epidemiology were concerned with the causes (etiology) of communicable diseases, and such work remains essential since it can lead to the identification of preventive methods. In this sense, epidemiology is a basic medical science with the goal of improving the health of populations.

The causation of some diseases can be linked exclusively to genetic factors, as with phenylketonuria, but is more commonly the result of an interaction between genetic and environmental factors. In this context, environment is defined broadly to include any biological, chemical, physical, psychological or other factors that can affect health (Chapter 9). Behaviour and lifestyle are of great importance in this connection, and epidemiology is increasingly used to study both their influence and preventive intervention through health promotion.

Epidemiology is also concerned with the course and outcome (natural history) of diseases in individuals and groups. The application of epidemiological principles and methods to problems encountered in the practice of medicine with individual patients has led to the development of clinical epidemiology. Epidemiology thus lends strong support to both preventive and clinical medicine.

Epidemiology is often used to describe the health status of population groups. Knowledge of the disease burden in populations is essential for health authorities, which seek to use limited resources to the best possible effect by

Fig. 1.2. Uses of epidemiology

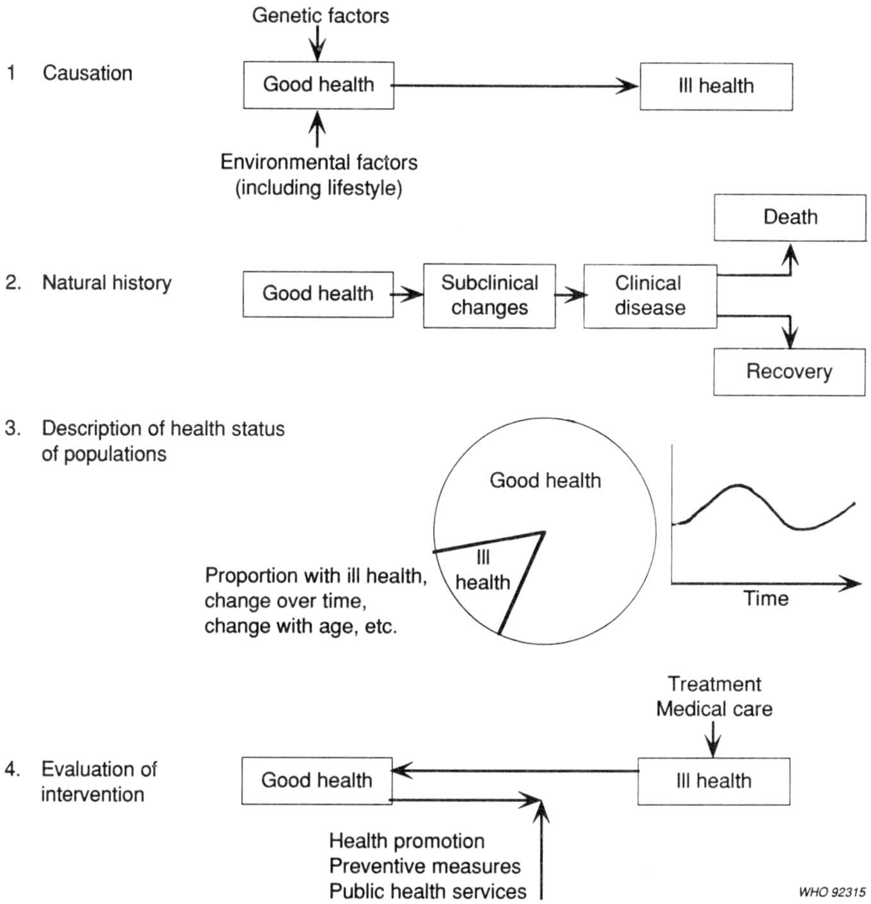

1 Causation
Genetic factors
Good health
Ill health
Environmental factors
(including lifestyle)

2. Natural history
Good health
Subclinical changes
Clinical disease
Death
Recovery

3. Description of health status of populations
Good health
Ill health
Proportion with ill health, change over time, change with age, etc.
Time

4. Evaluation of intervention
Treatment
Medical care
Good health
Ill health
Health promotion
Preventive measures
Public health services

WHO 92315

identifying priority health programmes for prevention and care. In some specialist areas, such as environmental and occupational epidemiology, the emphasis is on studies of populations with particular types of environmental exposure.

Recently, epidemiologists have become involved in evaluating the effectiveness and efficiency of health services, by determining the appropriate length of stay in hospital for specific conditions, the value of treating high blood pressure, the efficiency of sanitation measures to control diarrhoeal diseases, the impact on public health of reducing lead additives in petrol, and so on.

Achievements in epidemiology

Smallpox

The elimination of smallpox from the world contributed greatly to the health and well-being of millions of people, particularly in many of the poorest countries. It illustrates both the achievements and frustrations of modern public health. In the 1790s it was shown that cowpox infection conferred protection against the smallpox virus, yet it took almost 200 years for the benefits of this discovery to be accepted and applied throughout the world.

An intensive campaign to eliminate smallpox was coordinated over many years by WHO. Epidemiology played a central role by providing information about the distribution of cases and the model, mechanisms and levels of transmission, by mapping outbreaks of the disease, and by evaluating control measures. When a ten-year eradication programme was proposed by WHO in 1967, 10–15 million new cases and 2 million deaths were occurring annually in 31 countries. A very rapid reduction occurred in the number of countries reporting cases in the period 1967–76; by 1976 smallpox was reported from only two countries, and the last naturally occurring case of smallpox was reported in 1977 (Fig. 1.3). The outlay of approximately US$ 200 million has been estimated to result in savings of US$ 1500 million a year, mostly in the more affluent countries where vaccination programmes are no longer needed.

Fig. 1.3. Number of countries with smallpox, 1967–1978

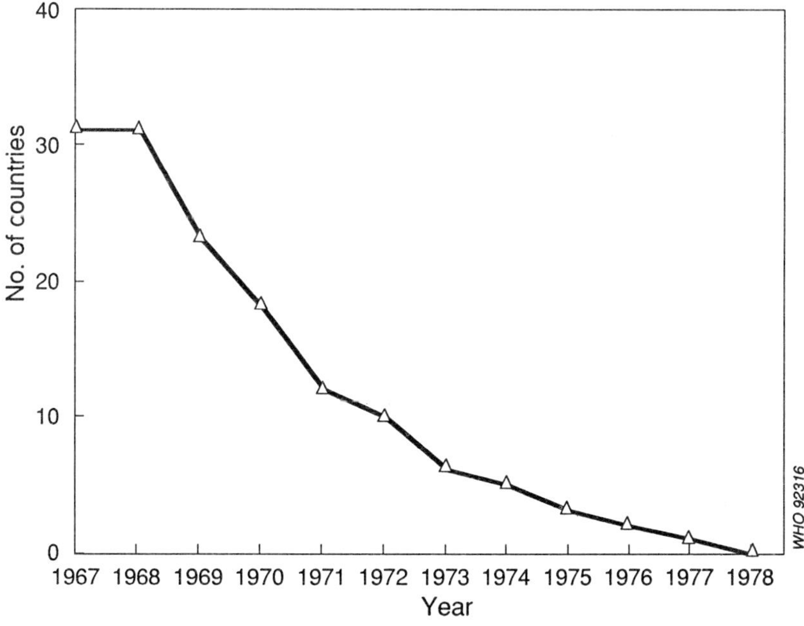

Source: Fenner et al., 1988.

Several factors contributed to the success of the programme: universal political commitment, a definite goal, a precise timetable, well trained staff and a flexible strategy. Furthermore, the disease had many features that made its elimination possible, and an effective heat-stable vaccine was available.

Methylmercury poisoning

Mercury was already known to be a hazardous substance in the Middle Ages. More recently it has become a symbol of the dangers of environmental pollution. In the 1950s, mercury compounds were released with the water discharged from a factory in Minamata, Japan, into a small bay. This led to the accumulation of methylmercury in fish, causing severe poisoning in people who ate them (WHO, 1976).

Epidemiology played a crucial role in identifying the cause and in the control of what was one of the first reported epidemics of disease caused by environmental pollution. The first cases were thought to be of infectious meningitis. However, it was observed that 121 patients with the disease mostly resided close to Minamata Bay. A survey of affected and unaffected people showed that the victims were almost exclusively members of families whose main occupation was fishing. People visiting these families and family members who ate small amounts of fish did not suffer from the disease. It was concluded that something in the fish had poisoned the patients and that the disease was not communicable or genetically determined.

This was the first known outbreak of methylmercury poisoning involving fish, and it took several years of research before the exact cause was identified. Minamata disease has become one of the best-documented environmental diseases. A second outbreak occurred in the 1960s in another part of Japan. Less severe poisoning from methylmercury in fish has since been reported from several other countries (WHO, 1990b).

Rheumatic fever and rheumatic heart disease

Rheumatic fever and rheumatic heart disease are associated with poverty, and in particular with poor housing and overcrowding, both of which favour the spread of streptococcal upper respiratory tract infections. In many developed countries, the decline in rheumatic fever started at the beginning of the twentieth century, long before the introduction of effective drugs such as sulfonamides and penicillin (Fig. 1.4). Today the disease has almost disappeared from developed countries although pockets of relatively high incidence still exist among socially and economically disadvantaged groups. In many developing countries, rheumatic heart disease is one of the most common forms of heart disease (WHO, 1988a).

Epidemiology has contributed to our understanding of the cause of rheumatic fever and rheumatic heart disease and to the development of methods for the prevention of rheumatic heart disease. Epidemiological studies have also highlighted the role of social and economic factors that contribute to outbreaks of rheumatic fever and to the spread of streptococcal throat infection. Clearly, the causation of these diseases is more complex than that of methylmercury poisoning, for which there is one specific causal factor.

Fig. 1.4. Reported rheumatic fever occurrence in Denmark, 1862–1962

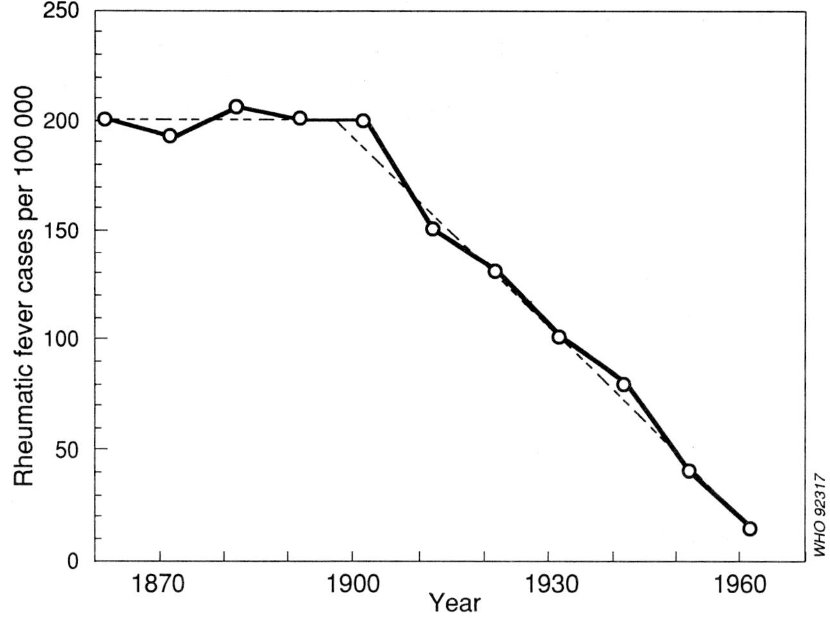

Source: Taranta & Markowitz, 1989. Reproduced by kind permission of the publisher.

Iodine deficiency diseases

Iodine deficiency, which occurs commonly in certain mountainous regions, causes loss of physical and mental energy associated with inadequate production of the iodine-containing thyroid hormone (Hetzel, 1989). Goitre and cretinism were first described in detail some 400 years ago, but it was not until the twentieth century that sufficient knowledge was acquired to permit effective prevention and control. In 1915, endemic goitre was named as the easiest known disease to prevent, and use of iodized salt for goitre control was proposed the same year in Switzerland (Hetzel, 1989). The first large-scale trials with iodine were carried out shortly afterwards in Akron, Ohio, USA, on 5000 girls aged between 11 and 18 years. The prophylactic and therapeutic effects were impressive and iodized salt was introduced on a community scale in many countries in 1924.

The use of iodized salt is effective because salt is used by all sections of society at roughly the same level throughout the year. Success depends on the effective production and distribution of the salt and requires legislative enforcement, quality control and public awareness.

Epidemiology has contributed to identifying and solving the iodine deficiency problem; effective measures of prevention suitable for use on a mass scale have been demonstrated, as have methods of monitoring iodization programmes. Nevertheless, there have been unnecessary delays in using this knowledge to reduce suffering among the millions of people in those developing countries where iodine deficiency is still endemic.

High blood pressure

High blood pressure (hypertension) is an important health problem in both developed and developing countries; up to 20% of people aged 35–64 years have hypertension in societies as diverse as those of the USA and parts of China. Epidemiology has defined the extent of the problem, established the natural history of the condition and the health consequences of untreated hypertension, demonstrated the value of treatment, and helped to determine the most appropriate blood pressure level at which treatment should begin. This level influences the number of people to be treated, and also allows an estimate of the costs of treatment. In the USA, for example, 53% of the white male population aged 65–74 would be defined as hypertensive according to current recommendations for treatment, whereas a more conservative cut-off point would mean that only 17% of this population would be regarded as hypertensive (Table 1.2). Hypertension is largely preventable, and epidemiological studies are central to the evaluation of preventive strategies.

Table 1.2. Proportion of US white males aged 65–74 years with raised blood pressure according to criteria for hypertension

Blood pressure (systolic/diastolic) (mm Hg)[a]	Percentage of population
⩾ 140/90	53
⩾ 160/95	24
⩾ 170/95	17

Source: Drizd et al., 1986.

[a] One or both of systolic and diastolic pressures.

Smoking, asbestos and lung cancer

Lung cancer used to be rare, but since the 1930s there has been a dramatic increase in the occurrence of the disease, particularly in industrialized countries. The first epidemiological studies linking lung cancer and smoking were published in 1950. Subsequent work has confirmed this association in a wide variety of populations. Many substances capable of causing cancer have been found in tobacco smoke.

It is now clear that the main cause of increasing lung cancer death rates is tobacco smoking (Fig. 1.1). There are, however, other causes such as asbestos dust and urban air pollution. Smoking and exposure to asbestos interact, creating exceedingly high lung cancer rates for workers who both smoke and are exposed to asbestos dust (Table 1.3).

Epidemiological studies can provide quantitative measurements of the contribution to disease causation of different environmental factors. The concept of causation is discussed in Chapter 5.

Table 1.3. Age-standardized lung cancer death rates (per 100 000 population) in relation to cigarette smoking and occupational exposure to asbestos dust

Exposure to asbestos	History of cigarette smoking	Lung cancer death rate per 100 000
No	No	11
Yes	No	58
No	Yes	123
Yes	Yes	602

Source: Hammond et al., 1979.

Hip fractures

Epidemiological research on injuries often involves collaboration between scientists in epidemiology and in the social and environmental health fields. Injuries related to falls, in particular fracture of the neck of the femur (hip fracture) in the elderly, have attracted a great deal of attention in recent years because of the implications for the health service needs of an aging population.

Of all injuries, hip fractures account for the largest number of days spent in hospital; the economic costs associated with hip fracture are considerable. Most hip fractures are the result of a fall, and most deaths associated with falls are the consequence of complications of fractures, especially in the elderly. Fractures in the elderly are associated with an increased tendency to fall, the intensity of trauma associated with falling and the ability of the bone to withstand trauma (Cummings & Nevitt, 1989). However, the relative importance of these influences is uncertain and, as a consequence, the optimal strategy to prevent hip fractures is unclear. The only area of general agreement is that the use of estrogen by postmenopausal women minimizes bone loss and has a part to play in the prevention of hip fracture in some women. Recent use (within two years) of estrogens appears to afford greater protection than earlier use, although the ideal duration and dose have not yet been established. The relevance of the findings to older women (over 75 years) cannot be determined as almost all epidemiological studies conducted to date have excluded that age group.

With the increasing number of elderly individuals in the population, the incidence of hip fracture can be expected to increase proportionately if efforts are not directed towards prevention. Epidemiology has a vital part to play in examining both modifiable and nonmodifiable factors in an effort to reduce the burden of such fractures.

AIDS

The acquired immunodeficiency syndrome (AIDS) was first identified as a distinct disease entity in 1981 in the USA (Gottlieb et al., 1981). By April 1992, 484 148 cases had been reported, some 45% in the USA, 13% in Europe, 30% in Africa, and 12% in Asia and other areas (WHO, 1992a).

The number of cases is likely to be much higher than that reported. The true extent of the problem is indicated by the number of people with AIDS-related conditions and the number infected with the causative human immunodeficiency virus (HIV) (Fig. 1.5).

Fig. 1.5. AIDS: the hidden epidemic

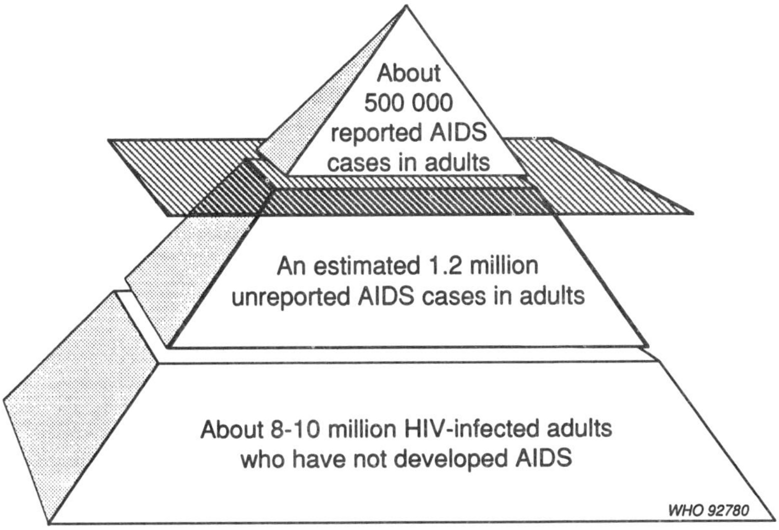

About 500 000 reported AIDS cases in adults

An estimated 1.2 million unreported AIDS cases in adults

About 8-10 million HIV-infected adults who have not developed AIDS

WHO 92780

Figures and estimates as of mid-1992.

Up to 50% of people diagnosed as having HIV infection are likely to develop the disease within ten years, and of those who get the disease more than 50% die within 18 months of diagnosis. In the USA, AIDS is already a more important cause of premature death than chronic obstructive lung disease and diabetes mellitus.

The virus is found in certain body fluids, particularly blood and seminal and uterovaginal fluids, and transmission occurs mainly through sexual intercourse or sharing of contaminated needles. The virus is also transmitted through transfusion of contaminated blood or blood products and from an infected woman to her offspring during pregnancy or at birth.

Full-blown AIDS causes a high mortality rate, although new, expensive drugs such as zidovudine (AZT) can have a delaying effect. Epidemiological studies have been vital in identifying the epidemic, determining the pattern of its spread, identifying risk factors, and evaluating interventions aimed at treating the disease and preventing and controlling the epidemic. Neither a fully effective drug nor a preventive vaccine has yet been developed. The screening of donated blood, the encouragement of safe sexual practices and the avoidance of needle-sharing are the main ways of controlling the spread of AIDS at present.

Study questions

1.1 Table 1.1 (page 1) indicates that there were over 40 times more cholera cases in one district than in another. Did this reflect the risk of catching cholera in each district?

1.2 How could the role of the water supply in causing deaths from cholera have been tested further?

1.3 Why do you suppose the study shown in Fig. 1.1 was restricted to doctors?

1.4 What conclusions can be drawn from Fig. 1.1?

1.5 Which factors need to be considered when interpreting geographical distributions of disease?

1.6 What changes occurred in the reported occurrence of rheumatic fever in Denmark during the period covered in Fig. 1.4? What might explain them?

1.7 What does Table 1.3 tell us about the contribution of asbestos exposure and smoking to the risk of lung cancer?

Chapter 2
Measuring health and disease

Definitions of health and disease

The most ambitious definition of health is that proposed by WHO in 1948: "health is a state of complete physical, mental, and social well-being and not merely the absence of disease or infirmity". This definition, although criticized because of the difficulty of defining and measuring well-being, remains an ideal. In 1977 the World Health Assembly resolved that the main target of Member States of WHO should be that by the year 2000 all people attain a level of health permitting them to lead socially and economically productive lives.

More practical definitions of health and disease are, of necessity, required; epidemiology concentrates on aspects of health that are relatively easily measurable and are priorities for action. In communities where progress has been made on the prevention of premature death and disability, increased attention is being devoted to positive health states. For example, a major new international initiative in health promotion was heralded by the 1986 Ottawa Charter (see Chapter 10).

Definitions of health states used by epidemiologists tend to be simple, e.g. "disease present" or "disease absent". The development of criteria to establish the presence of a disease requires definition of normality and abnormality. However, it is often difficult to define what is normal, and there is often no clear distinction between normal and abnormal.

Diagnostic criteria are usually based on symptoms, signs and test results. Thus hepatitis can be identified by the presence of antibodies in the blood, asbestosis by symptoms and signs of specific changes in lung function, radiographic demonstration of fibrosis of the lung tissue or pleural thickening, and a history of exposure to asbestos fibres. Table 2.1 shows a more complex example, the modified Jones diagnostic criteria for rheumatic fever proposed by the American Heart Association. A diagnosis can be made on the basis of several of the manifestations of the disease, some signs being more important than others.

In some situations very simple criteria are justified. For example, the reduction of mortality due to bacterial pneumonia in children in developing countries depends on rapid detection and treatment. WHO's case-management guidelines recommend that pneumonia case detection be based on clinical signs alone, without auscultation, chest X-rays or laboratory diagnostic tests. The only equipment required is a simple device for timing respiratory rate. The use of antibiotics for suspected pneumonia, based only on a physical examination, is justified in settings where there is a significant rate of bacterial pneumonia (WHO, 1993).

Table 2.1. The Jones criteria (revised) for guidance in the diagnosis of acute rheumatic fever

A high probability of rheumatic fever is indicated by the presence of two major, or one major and two minor, manifestations, if supported by evidence of a preceding Group A streptococcal infection.

Major manifestations	Minor manifestations
Carditis	*Clinical:*
Polyarthritis	fever
Chorea	arthralgia (joint pains)
Erythema marginatum	previous rheumatic fever or rheumatic heart disease
Subcutaneous nodules	
	Laboratory:
	acute-phase reactants:
	abnormal erythrocyte sedimentation rate, C-reactive protein, leukocytosis
	prolonged P-R interval

Source: WHO, 1988a.

A clinical case definition for AIDS in adults, developed in 1985 and later revised (WHO, 1986), refers to the existence of at least two major signs in association with at least one minor sign, in the absence of other known causes of suppression of the immune system, such as cancer or severe malnutrition. This definition has been tested in Zaire and found to be reliable (Colebunders et al., 1987).

Diagnostic criteria may change quite rapidly as knowledge increases or techniques improve. For example, the original WHO criteria for myocardial infarction, for use in epidemiological studies, have been modified by the introduction of an objective method, the Minnesota Code, for assessing electrocardiograms (Prineas et al., 1982).

Whatever the definitions used in epidemiology, it is essential that they be clearly stated, easy to use and easy to measure in a standard manner under a wide variety of circumstances by different people. Definitions used in clinical practice are less rigidly specified and clinical judgement is more important in diagnosis, at least partly because it is often possible to proceed stepwise with a series of tests until a diagnosis is confirmed. Epidemiological studies may use data from clinical practice but are often based on data collected for the early detection of disease. The principles are described in Chapter 6 and, for instance, in a WHO publication on early detection of occupational disease (WHO, 1987c).

Measures of disease frequency

Population at risk

Several measures of disease frequency are based on the fundamental concepts of prevalence and incidence. Unfortunately, epidemiologists have not yet reached complete agreement on the definitions of terms used in this field. In this text we generally use the terms as defined in the *Dictionary of epidemiology* (Last, 1988).

It is important to note that the calculation of measures of disease frequency depends on correct estimates of the numbers of people under consideration. Ideally these figures should include only people who are potentially susceptible to the diseases studied. Clearly, for instance, men should not be included in calculations of the frequency of carcinoma of the cervix.

That part of a population which is susceptible to a disease is called the population at risk (Fig. 2.1). It can be defined on the basis of demographic or environmental factors. For instance, occupational injuries occur only among working people so the population at risk is the workforce; in some countries, brucellosis occurs only among people handling infected animals so the population at risk consists of those working on farms and in slaughterhouses.

Fig. 2.1. Population at risk in a study of carcinoma of the cervix

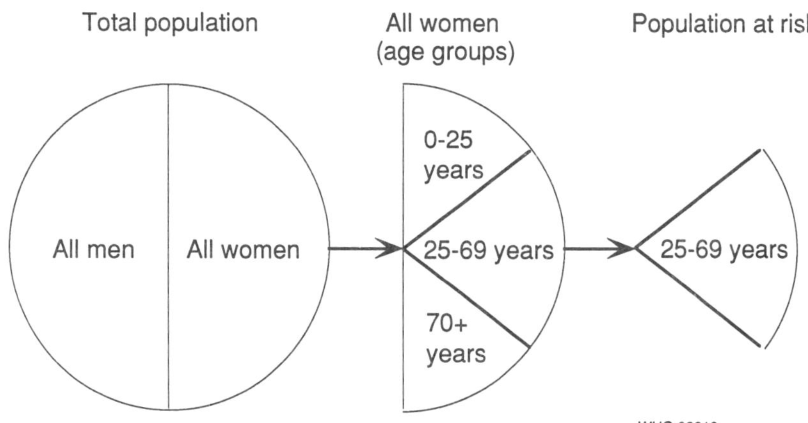

Prevalence and incidence

The prevalence of a disease is the number of cases in a defined population at a specified point in time, while its incidence is the number of new cases arising in a given period in a specified population. These are fundamentally different ways of measuring occurrence and the relation between prevalence and incidence varies between diseases. There may be a high prevalence and low incidence, as for diabetes, or a low prevalence and high incidence, as for the common cold; colds occur more frequently than diabetes but last only a short time, whereas once contracted diabetes is permanent.

Measuring prevalence and incidence basically involves the counting of cases in defined populations at risk. The number of cases alone without reference to the population at risk can occasionally give an impression of the overall magnitude of a health problem, or of short-term trends in a population, for instance during an epidemic. WHO's *Weekly epidemiological record* contains incidence data in the form of case numbers, which, in spite of their crude nature, can give useful information about the development of epidemics of communicable diseases, as with cholera and dengue.

Data on prevalence and incidence become much more useful if converted into rates (see Table 1.1, page 1). A rate is calculated by dividing the number of cases by the corresponding number of people in the population at risk, and is expressed as cases per 10^n people. Some epidemiologists use the term "rate" only for measurements of disease occurrence per time unit (week, year, etc.). However, with this definition only incidence rate would be a true rate. In this text we use the more traditional definition of rate.

Prevalence rate

The prevalence rate (P) for a disease is calculated as follows:

$$P = \frac{\text{Number of people with the disease or condition at a specified time}}{\text{Number of people in the population at risk at the specified time}} \; (\times 10^n)$$

Data on the population at risk are not always available and in many studies the total population in the study area is used as an approximation.

The prevalence rate is often expressed as cases per 1000 or per 100 population. In this case, P has to be multiplied by the appropriate factor 10^n. If the data have been collected for one point in time, P is the "point prevalence rate". It is sometimes more convenient to use the "period prevalence rate", calculated as the total number of persons known to have had a disease or attribute at any time during a specified period, divided by the population at risk of having the disease or attribute midway through the period.

Several factors can influence prevalence rate. In particular:

- the severity of illness (if many people who develop a disease die its prevalence rate is depressed);
- the duration of illness (if a disease lasts a short time its prevalence rate is lower than if it lasts a long time);
- the number of new cases (if many people develop a disease its prevalence rate is higher than if few people do so);

A summary of factors influencing observed prevalence rates is given in Fig. 2.2.

Since prevalence rates are influenced by so many factors unrelated to disease causation, prevalence studies do not usually provide strong evidence of causality. Measures of prevalence rate are, however, helpful in assessing the need for health care and the planning of health services. Prevalence rates are often used to measure the occurrence of conditions for which the onset of disease may be gradual, such as maturity-onset diabetes or rheumatoid arthritis. The prevalence rate of non-insulin-dependent diabetes mellitus has been measured in various populations using criteria proposed by WHO (Table 2.2); it varies greatly, suggesting the importance of factors related to country or ethnic background in causing this disease and indicating the varying need for diabetic health services in different populations.

Fig. 2.2. Factors influencing observed prevalence rate

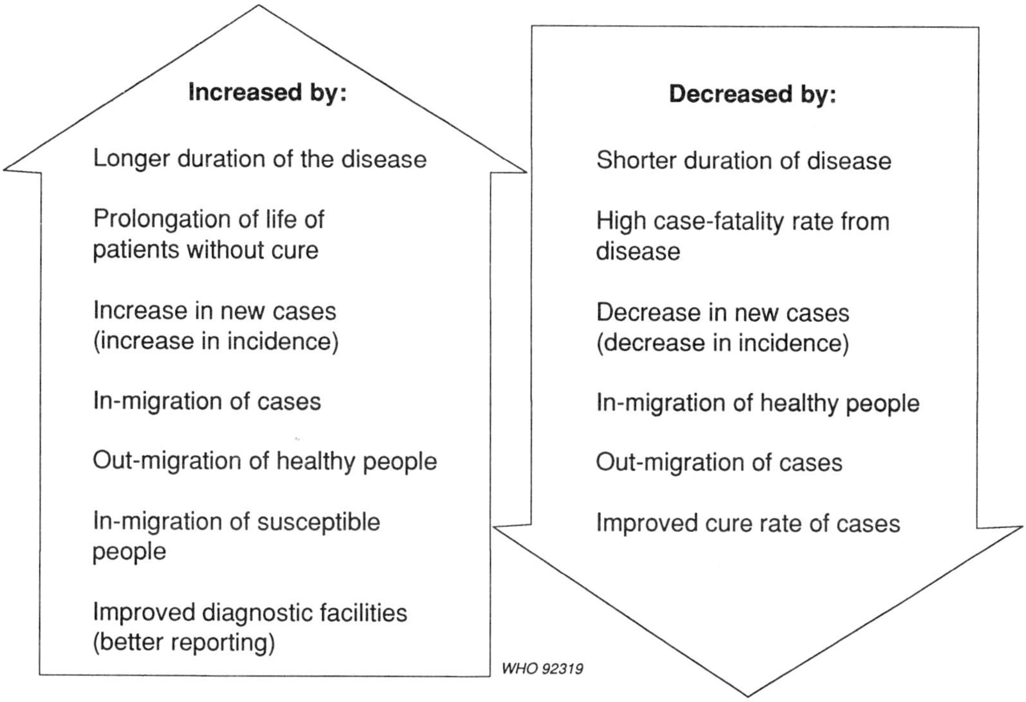

Table 2.2. Prevalence rate of non-insulin-dependent diabetes mellitus in selected populations

Location/population	Age group (years)	Prevalence rate (%)
Fiji Indians	20 +	13.5
Indonesia	15 +	1.7
Israel	40–70	15.9
Malta	15 +	7.7
Mexican Americans (USA)	25–64	17.0
Nauru	20 +	24.3
Pima Indians (USA)	25 +	25.5
USA	20–74	6.9

Source: WHO, 1985.

Incidence rate

In the calculation of incidence rates the numerator is the number of new events that occur in a defined time period and the denominator is the population at risk of experiencing the event during this period. The most accurate way of calculating incidence rate is to calculate what Last (1988) calls "person-time incidence rate". Each person in the study population contributes one person-year to the denominator for each year of observation before disease develops or the person is lost to follow-up.

Incidence rate (I) is calculated as follows:

$$I = \frac{\text{Number of people who get a disease in a specified period}}{\text{Sum of the length of time during which each person in the population is at risk}} (\times 10^n)$$

The numerator strictly refers only to first events of disease. The units of incidence rate must always include a dimension of time (day, month, year, etc.).

For each individual in the population, the time at risk is that during which the person under observation remains disease-free. The denominator for the calculation of incidence rate is the sum of all the disease-free time periods in the defined time period of the study.

The incidence rate takes into account the variable time periods during which individuals are disease-free and thus at risk of developing the disease. Since it may not be possible to measure disease-free periods precisely, the denominator is often calculated approximately by multiplying the average size of the study population by the length of the study period. This is reasonably accurate if the size of the population is stable and the incidence rate is low.

In a study in the USA, the incidence rate of stroke was measured in 118 539 women who were 30–55 years of age and free from coronary heart disease, stroke and cancer in 1976 (Table 2.3). A total of 274 stroke cases were identified in the eight years of follow-up (908 447 person–years). The overall stroke incidence rate was 30.2 per 100 000 person–years of observation; the rate was higher for smokers than nonsmokers; that for ex-smokers was intermediate.

Table 2.3. Relationship between cigarette smoking and incidence rate of stroke in a cohort of 118 539 women

Smoking category	No. of cases of stroke	Person–years of observation (over 8 years)	Stroke incidence rate (per 100 000 person–years)
Never smoked	70	395 594	17.7
Ex-smoker	65	232 712	27.9
Smoker	139	280 141	49.6
Total	274	908 447	30.2

Source: Colditz et al., 1988. Reproduced by kind permission of the publisher.

Cumulative incidence rate or risk

Cumulative incidence rate is a simpler measure of the occurrence of a disease or health status. Unlike incidence rate, it measures the denominator only at the beginning of a study.

Cumulative incidence rate (*CI*) can be calculated as follows:

$$CI = \frac{\text{Number of people who get a disease during a specified period}}{\text{Number of people free of the disease in the population at risk at the beginning of the period}} (\times 10^n)$$

Cumulative incidence rate is often presented as cases per 1000 population. With reference again to Table 2.3, the cumulative incidence for stroke over the eight-year follow-up was 2.3 per 1000 (274 cases of stroke divided by the 118 539 women who entered the study). In a statistical sense the cumulative incidence is the probability or risk of individuals in the population getting the disease during the specified period.

The period can be of any length but is usually several years or even the whole life-time. The cumulative incidence rate therefore is similar to the "risk of death" concept used in actuarial and life-table calculations. Cumulative incidence rates have a simplicity that makes them suitable for the communication of health information to decision-makers. For instance, the statistics for deaths of men in Japan and Sri Lanka due to accidents and violence can be compared using annual death rates for each five-year age group as given in *World health statistics annual 1989* (WHO, 1990a). For each age group the rates are higher in Sri Lanka than in Japan, but the differences vary. If we calculate the cumulative death rate in the age range 15–59, we find that the risk of a 15-year-old Japanese male dying an accidental or violent death is 28 per 1000, whereas for a Sri Lankan of the same age the risk is 73 per 1000. These numbers are relatively easy to interpret and they provide a useful summary measure, the mortality risk or cumulative mortality rate, for comparing health risks in different populations.

Case–fatality

Case–fatality is a measure of the severity of a disease and is defined as the proportion of cases of a specified disease or condition which are fatal within a specified time.

$$\text{Case–fatality (\%)} = \frac{\text{Number of deaths from a disease in a specified period}}{\text{Number of diagnosed cases of the disease in the same period}} \times 100$$

This is, strictly speaking, the fatality/case ratio, but is often called the case–fatality rate.

Interrelationships of the different measures

Prevalence rate is dependent on both incidence rate and disease duration. Provided that the prevalence rate (*P*) is low and does not vary significantly with time, it can be calculated approximately as:

$$P = \text{incidence rate} \times \text{average duration of disease}$$

The cumulative incidence rate of a disease depends on both the incidence rate and the length of the period of interest. Since the incidence rate usually changes with age, age-specific incidence rates often have to be considered. The cumulative incidence rate is a useful approximation of incidence rate when the rate is low or when the study period is short.

Let us consider the various measures of disease occurrence in a hypothetical example of seven people investigated for seven years. In Fig. 2.3 it can be seen that:

- the incidence rate of the disease during the seven-year period is the number of new events (3) divided by the sum of the lengths of time at risk of getting the disease for the population (33 person-years), i.e. 9.1 cases per 100 person-years;
- the cumulative incidence rate is the number of new events (3) divided by the number of people at risk free of the disease at the beginning of the period (7), i.e. 43 cases per 100 persons during the seven years;
- the average duration of disease is the total number of years of disease divided by the number of cases, i.e. 10/3 = 3.3 years;

Fig. 2.3. Example of calculation of disease occurrence

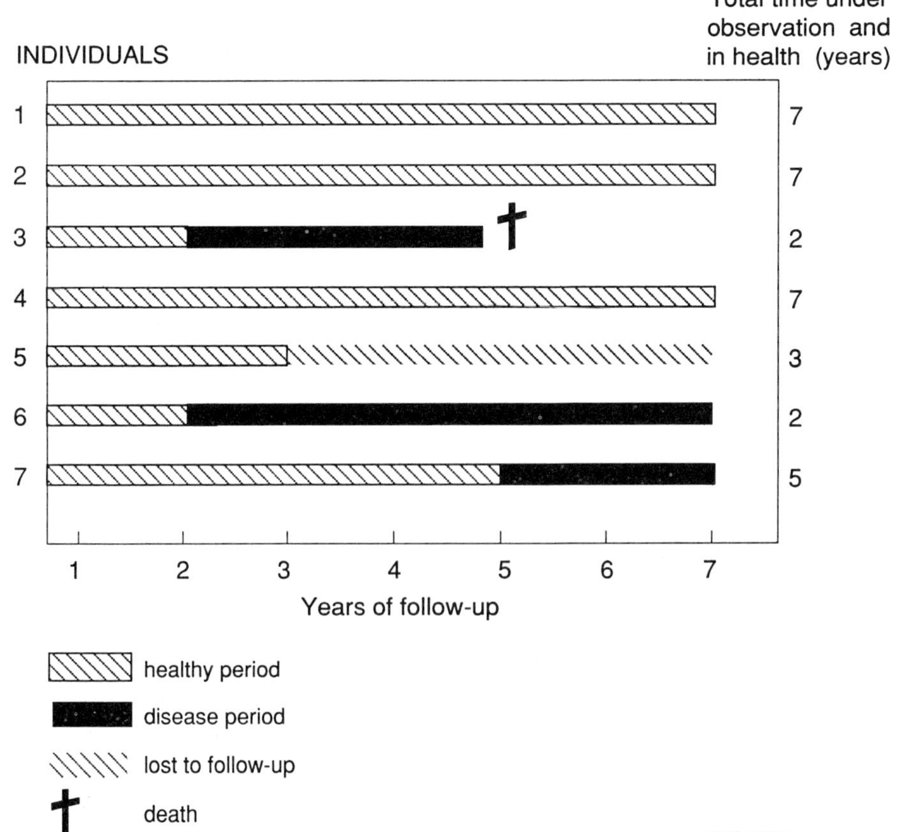

- the prevalence rate depends on the point in time at which the study takes place; at the start of year 4, for example, it is the ratio of the number of people with the disease (2) to the number of people in the population observed at that time (6), i.e. 33 cases per 100 persons.
- the formula given on page 19 for prevalence rate would give an estimated average prevalence of 30 cases per 100 population (9.1×3.3).

Use of available information

Mortality

Epidemiologists often begin the investigation of the health experience of a population with information that is routinely available. In many countries the fact and cause of death are recorded on a standard death certificate, which also carries information on age, sex, date of birth and place of residence. The data are open to various sources of error but, from an epidemiological perspective, often provide invaluable information on trends in a population's health status. The usefulness of the data depends on many factors, including the completeness of records and the accuracy with which the underlying causes of death are assigned, especially in elderly people for whom autopsy rates are often low.

Unfortunately, in many countries basic mortality statistics are not yet available, usually because resources do not permit the establishment of routine death registers. Where national registers exist they may not be complete; poorer segments of populations may not be covered, deaths may not be reported for cultural or religious reasons, and the age at death may not be given accurately. The provision of accurate death data is a priority for epidemiologists.

Internationally agreed classification procedures, which are given in the *International classification of diseases* (WHO, 1992b) and revised at regular intervals to take account of the emergence of new diseases and changes in criteria for established diseases, are used for coding causes of death. The data are expressed as death rates. The coding of causes of death is quite complex and is not yet a matter of routine in all countries.

The death rate or crude mortality rate is calculated as follows:

$$\text{Crude mortality rate} = \frac{\text{Number of deaths in a specified period}}{\text{Average total population during that period}} (\times 10^n)$$

The main disadvantage of the crude mortality rate is that it takes no account of the fact that the chance of dying varies according to age, sex, race, socio-economic class, and other factors. It is usually not appropriate to use it for comparing different time periods or geographical areas. For example, patterns of death among residents in newly occupied urban developments with many young families are likely to be very different from those in seaside resorts where many retired people choose to live. Comparisons of mortality rates between groups of diverse age structure are usually based on age-standardized rates (see page 25).

Death rates can be usefully expressed for specific groups in a population which are defined by age, race, sex, occupation or geographical location, or for specific causes of death. For example, an age- and sex-specific death rate is defined as follows:

$$\frac{\text{Total number of deaths occurring in a specific age- and sex-group of the population in a defined area during a specified period}}{\text{Estimated total population of the same age- and sex-group of the population in the same area during the same period}} (\times 10^n)$$

Occasionally the mortality in a population is described by using the proportionate mortality rate, which is actually a ratio: the number of deaths from a given cause per 100 or 1000 total deaths in the same period.

A proportionate rate does not express the risk of members of a population contracting or dying from a disease. Comparisons of proportionate rates between groups may suggest interesting differences. However, unless the crude or group-specific mortality rates are known it cannot be clear whether a difference between groups relates to variations in the numerators or the denominators. For example, proportionate mortality rates for cancer are much greater in typical developed countries with many old people than in developing countries with few old people, even if the actual lifetime risk of cancer is the same.

Mortality before and just after birth

The infant mortality rate is commonly used as an indicator of the level of health in a community. It measures the death rate in children during the first year of life, the denominator being the number of live births in the same year.

The infant mortality rate is calculated as follows:

$$\text{Infant mortality rate} = \frac{\text{Number of deaths in a year of children less than 1 year of age}}{\text{Number of live births in the same year}} \times 1000$$

The use of infant mortality rates as a measure of overall health status for a given population is based on the assumption that it is particularly sensitive to socioeconomic changes and to health-care interventions. Infant mortality rates vary enormously (see Table 2.4). High rates should alert health professionals to the need for investigation and preventive action on a broad front.

Other measures of mortality in early childhood include the fetal death rate, the stillbirth or late fetal death rate, the perinatal mortality rate, the neonatal mortality rate, and the postneonatal mortality rate. Precise guidelines on the definition of stillbirth, fetal death and live birth can be found in *International classification of diseases* (WHO, 1992b) and *Teaching health statistics* (Lwanga & Tye, 1986).

The child mortality rate is based on deaths of children aged 1–4 years and is important because accidental injuries, malnutrition and infectious diseases are common in this age group.

Table 2.4. Infant mortality rates in selected countries, 1987

Country	Infant mortality rate (per 1000 live births)
Japan	4.8
Sweden	6.1
Switzerland	6.8
Canada	7.3
France	7.8
Australia	8.7
England and Wales	9.0
USA	10.1
Portugal	13.1
Cuba	13.3
Hungary	15.8
Poland	16.2
Chile	18.5
Fiji	19.8
Yugoslavia	25.1
Ecuador	47.7
Morocco[a]	90
Bangladesh[a]	124
Ethiopia[a]	152
Afghanistan[a]	189

Source: WHO, 1990a.
[a] Figures estimated by UNICEF (1987).

Where accurate death registers do not exist, infant and child mortality can be estimated from information collected in household surveys in which the following question is asked initially:

> "During the last two years, have any children died who were aged five years or less?"

If the answer is in the affirmative, three more questions are put:

> "How many months ago did the death occur?"
>
> "How many months of age was the child at death?"
>
> "Was the child a boy or a girl?"

If information on the number and ages of surviving children is also collected during a survey, infant and child mortality rates can be estimated reasonably accurately. Adult mortality can be measured approximately in household surveys if accurate information is not already available.

There are problems with household surveys. In particular, respondents may not understand the time span of the question, children who die shortly after birth may be left out, and for cultural reasons more male deaths than female deaths may be reported. However, this is the only method that is applicable in some communities. Measurement of infant mortality in low-income communities is particularly important in helping planners to address the need for equity in health care. In the absence of reliable data, the extent of health problems may not be recognized. Details on the method can be found in the *Handbook of household surveys* (United Nations, 1984) or in *Asking demographic questions* (Lucas & Kane, 1985).

The maternal mortality rate, an important statistic that may be neglected because it is difficult to calculate accurately, is given by:

$$\text{Maternal mortality rate} = \frac{\text{Maternal pregnancy-related deaths in one year}}{\text{Total births in same year}} (\times 10^n)$$

The maternal mortality rate varies enormously from about 10 per 100 000 in Europe to over 500 per 100 000 in Africa. Even this comparison does not adequately reflect the much greater risk of dying from pregnancy-related causes in Africa. The average number of births per woman is also higher in Africa, and the risk of a woman dying from pregnancy-related causes may be about 400 times greater in some developing countries than in developed countries.

Life expectancy

Life expectancy is another frequently used summary measure of the health status of a population. It is defined as the average number of years an individual of a given age is expected to live if current mortality rates continue. It is not always easy to interpret the reasons for the differences in life expectancy between countries; different patterns may emerge according to the measures that are used. Life expectancy at birth, as an overall measure of health status, attaches greater importance to deaths in infancy than to deaths later in life. Table 2.5 gives data for four countries with reasonably accurate mortality statistics. In the least developed countries the life expectancy at birth may be as low as 40–50 years.

Table 2.5. Life expectancy (years) at selected ages for four countries

Age	Mauritius	Bulgaria	USA	Japan
Birth	65.0	68.3	71.6	75.8
45 years	25.3	27.3	30.4	32.9
65 years	11.7	12.6	15.0	16.2

Source: WHO, 1990a.

Other measures of health status based on mortality data have been proposed. One, years of potential life lost, is based on the years of life lost through premature death (before an arbitrarily determined age). More complex measures take into account not only the duration of life but also some notion of its quality, e.g. life expectancy free from disability, and quality-adjusted life years; the latter are increasingly used in estimates of the cost-effectiveness of various procedures, as described in Chapter 10.

A method has been developed by the Ghana Health Assessment Project Team (1981) to assess quantitatively the relative importance of different disease problems for the health of a population. The method measures the impact of a disease on a community by the number of days of healthy life lost through illness, disability and death as a consequence of the disease. This measure is derived by combining information on incidence rate, case-fatality and the extent and duration of disability produced by the disease. In Ghana it has been estimated that malaria, measles, childhood pneumonia, sickle cell anaemia and severe malnutrition are the five most important causes of loss of healthy life, and between them they account for 34% of healthy life lost due to diseases.

Standardized rates

An age-standardized death rate (sometimes referred to as an age-adjusted rate) is a summary measure of the death rate that a population would have if it had a standard age structure. Standardization is necessary when comparing two or more populations that differ with respect to some basic characteristics (age, race, socioeconomic status, etc.) that independently influence the risk of death. Two frequently used standard populations are the Segi world population and the European standard population (WHO, 1990a). The standardization of rates can be done either directly or indirectly. The indirect method is the more frequently used, whereby the disease rates in the standard population are applied to the populations being compared. This procedure yields the number of cases that would be expected if the age-specific rates in the standard population were true for the study population. The choice of a standard population is arbitrary. Details on methods of standardizing rates can be found in Lwanga & Tye (1986). Standardized rates are used, whenever relevant, for morbidity as well as mortality.

The age-standardization of rates eliminates the influence of different age distributions on the morbidity or mortality rates being compared. For example, there is great variation between countries in the reported crude mortality rates for diseases of the circulatory system (Table 2.6). Finland has a crude rate approximately five times that of Mexico, but the standardized rate is less than twice as high. Egypt has the highest age-standardized rate and the highest age-specific rates in Table 2.6, even though the crude rate is less than half that of

Table 2.6. Crude and age-standardized mortality rates (per 100 000) for diseases of the circulatory system in selected countries, 1980

	Crude rate	Standardized rate, all ages	Age-specific rate	
			45–54 years	55–64 years
Finland	491	277	204	631
New Zealand	369	254	184	559
France	368	164	97	266
Japan	247	154	95	227
Egypt	192	299	301	790
Venezuela	115	219	177	497
Mexico	95	163	132	327

Calculated from data in WHO, 1987a.

Finland. Thus the difference between these countries is not as large as it appears from the crude rates. Developing countries have a much greater proportion of young people in their populations than do developed countries, and the young have low rates of cardiovascular disease compared with older people. All these rates are, of course, influenced by the quality of the original data on causes of death.

Whereas in Table 2.6 standardization is done for the complete age range, in Table 2.7 only the range 30–69 years is covered. The mortality rates for coronary heart disease and stroke are standardized to a part of a standard population (Segi world population) to ensure that the comparisons are not influenced by the different age distributions in the various populations. Table 2.7 shows large variations in the rates and great differences between men and women, particularly for coronary heart disease.

Table 2.7. Age-standardized mortality rates (per 100 000) in the 30–69-year age group, for coronary heart disease and stroke

	Coronary heart disease		Stroke	
	Men	Women	Men	Women
Northern Ireland	406	130	62	50
Scotland	398	142	73	57
Finland	390	79	74	43
Czechoslovakia	346	101	130	75
England and Wales	318	94	52	40
New Zealand	296	94	46	38
Australia	247	76	44	33
United States of America	235	80	34	26
Poland	230	54	72	47
Greece	135	33	60	44
Portugal	104	32	20	74
France	94	20	45	21
Japan	38	13	79	45

Source: Uemura & Pisa, 1988.

Morbidity

Death rates are particularly useful for investigating diseases with a high case–fatality. However, many diseases have low case–fatality, e.g. varicose veins, rheumatoid arthritis, chickenpox and mumps. In this situation, data on morbidity (the frequency of illness) are more useful than mortality rates. Morbidity data are often helpful in clarifying the reasons for particular trends in mortality. Changes in death rates could be due to changes in morbidity rates or in case-fatality. For example, the recent decline in cardiovascular disease mortality rates in many developed countries could be due to a fall in either incidence or case–fatality. Because population age structures change with time, time-trend analysis should be based on age-standardized morbidity and mortality rates.

In many countries some morbidity data are collected to meet legal requirements, e.g. in respect of notifiable diseases. Quarantinable diseases, such as cholera, and other serious communicable diseases, such as Lassa fever and AIDS, are often included among the notifiable diseases. Notification depends on patients seeking medical advice, the correct diagnosis being made, and the notifications being forwarded to the public health authorities; many cases may never be notified. For diseases of major public health importance, notifications are collated by WHO and published in the *Weekly epidemiological record.*

Other sources of information on morbidity are data on hospital admissions and discharges, outpatient and primary health care consultations, and specialist services (such as accident treatment), and registers of disease events such as cancer and congenital malformations. To be useful for epidemiological studies the data must be relevant and easily accessible. In some countries the confidential nature of medical records may render hospital data inaccessible for epidemiological studies. A recording system focusing on administrative or financial data, rather than on diagnostic and individual characteristics, may diminish the epidemiological value of routine health service data.

Hospital admission rates are influenced by factors other than the morbidity of the population, among them the availability of beds, admission policies and social factors. The dramatic rise in hospital admission rates for asthma in young children in New Zealand between 1960 and 1980, for example, may have many possible explanations including changes in incidence rates and admission policies (Table 2.8). If hospital admission events rather than individuals are recorded, it may not be possible to separate first admissions from readmissions. The population served by a hospital (the denominator) may prove difficult to determine.

Table 2.8. Hospital admission rates for asthma per 100 000 by age (Auckland, New Zealand)

	Year		
Age group (years)	**1960**	**1970**	**1980**
0–14	40	160	450
15–44	45	115	200
45–64	70	115	220

Source: Jackson & Mitchell, 1983. Reproduced by kind permission of the publisher.

Because of the numerous limitations of routinely recorded morbidity data, many epidemiological studies of morbidity rely on the collection of new data using specially designed questionnaires and screening methods. This enables investigators to have more confidence in the data and the rates calculated from them.

Disability

To an increasing extent, measurements concern not only the occurrence of diseases, as with incidence and morbidity rates, but also the persistence of the consequences of disease: impairments, disabilities and handicaps. These have been defined by WHO as follows (WHO, 1980b):

impairment: any loss or abnormality of psychological, physiological or anatomical structure or function;

disability: any restriction or lack (resulting from an impairment) of ability to perform an activity in the manner or within the range considered normal for a human being;

handicap: a disadvantage for a given individual, resulting from an impairment or a disability, that limits or prevents the fulfilment of a role that is normal (depending on age, sex, and social and cultural factors) for that individual.

Measurement of the prevalence of disability presents formidable problems and, even more than for morbidity, is affected by extraneous social factors. It is, however, becoming increasingly important in societies where acute morbidity and fatal illness are decreasing and where there is an increasing number of aged people.

Comparing disease occurrence

Measuring the occurrence of disease or other health states is only the beginning of the epidemiological process. The next essential step is the comparison of occurrence in two or more groups of people whose exposures have differed. In a qualitative sense, an individual can be either exposed or unexposed to a factor under study. An unexposed group is often used as a reference group. In a quantitative sense, exposed people can have different levels and durations of exposure (see Chapter 9). The total amount of a factor that has reached an individual is called the dose.

The process of comparing occurrences can be used to calculate the risk that a health effect will result from an exposure. Both absolute and relative comparisons can be made; the measures describe the strength of an association between exposure and outcome.

Absolute comparison

Risk difference

The risk difference, also called attributable risk (exposed), excess risk or absolute risk, is the difference in rates of occurrence between exposed and unexposed groups. It is a useful measure of the extent of the public health problem caused by the exposure. For example, from the data in Table 2.3, the risk difference in respect of the stroke incidence rate for women who smoke compared with that for women who have never smoked is 31.9 per 100 000 person–years (49.6 – 17.7).

Attributable fraction (exposed)

The attributable fraction (exposed) or etiological fraction (exposed) is determined by dividing the risk difference by the rate of occurrence among the exposed population. For the data in Table 2.3 the attributable fraction of smoking for stroke in the women smokers is $((49.6 - 17.7)/49.6) \times 100 = 64\%$.

When an exposure is believed to be a cause of a given disease, the attributable fraction is the proportion of the disease in the specific population that would be eliminated in the absence of exposure. In the above example, one would expect to achieve a 64% reduction in the risk of stroke among the women smokers if smoking were stopped, on the assumption that smoking is both causal and preventable. Attributable fraction is a useful tool for assessing priorities for public health action. For example, both smoking and air pollution are causes of lung cancer, but the attributable fraction due to smoking is usually much greater than that due to air pollution. Only in communities with very low smoking prevalence and severe indoor or outdoor air pollution is the latter likely to be the major cause of lung cancer. In most countries, smoking control should take priority in lung cancer prevention programmes.

Population attributable risk

The population attributable risk or attributable fraction (population) is a measure of the excess rate of disease in a total study population which is attributable to an exposure. This measure is useful for determining the relative importance of exposures for the entire population and is the proportion by which the incidence rate of the outcome in the entire population would be reduced if exposure were eliminated. It may be estimated by the formula

$$AF_p = \frac{I_p - I_u}{I_p}$$

where I_p is the incidence rate of the disease in the total population and I_u is the incidence rate of the disease among the unexposed group.

From the data in Table 2.3, the population attributable risk or attributable fraction (population) is calculated as

$$\frac{30.2 - 17.7}{30.2} = 0.414$$

corresponding to 41.4%.

Relative comparison

The risk ratio or relative risk is the ratio of the risk of occurrence of a disease among exposed people to that among the unexposed. The risk ratio of stroke in women who smoke compared with those who have never smoked is 2.8 (49.6/17.7) (Table 2.3).

The risk ratio is a better indicator of the strength of an association than the risk difference, because it is expressed relative to a baseline level of occurrence. It is thus related to the magnitude of the baseline incidence rate, unlike the risk difference; populations with similar risk differences can have greatly differing risk ratios, depending on the magnitude of the baseline rates. The risk ratio is used in assessing the likelihood that an association represents a causal relationship. For example, the risk ratio of lung cancer in long-term heavy smokers compared with nonsmokers is approximately 20. This is very high and indicates that this relationship is not likely to be a chance finding. Of course, smaller risk ratios can also indicate a causal relationship, but care must be taken to eliminate other possible explanations (see Chapter 5).

The standardized mortality ratio is a special type of risk ratio in which the observed mortality pattern in a group is compared with what would have been expected if the age-specific mortality rates had been the same as in a specified reference population. The procedure, called indirect standardization, adjusts for differences in age distribution between the study and reference populations.

Study questions

2.1 What are the three epidemiological measures of disease frequency and how are they related?

2.2 Is prevalence rate a useful measure of the frequency of non-insulin-dependent diabetes in different populations? What are the possible explanations for the variation in diabetes prevalence rates indicated in Table 2.2?

2.3 Why have the coronary heart disease death rates in Table 2.7 been standardized for age? What are the possible explanations for the variation shown in the table?

2.4 What measures are used to compare the frequency of disease in populations and what information do they provide?

2.5 The relative risk of lung cancer associated with passive smoking is low, but the population attributable risk is considerable. What is the explanation for this?

Chapter 3
Types of study

Observations and experiments

Epidemiological studies can be classified as either observational or experimental. The most commonly used types of study are listed in Table 3.1 together with their units of study and their alternative names. The terms given in the left-hand column are used throughout this publication.

Table 3.1. Types of epidemiological study

Type of study	Alternative name	Unit of study
Observational studies		
Descriptive studies		
Analytical studies		
Ecological	Correlational	Populations
Cross-sectional	Prevalence	Individuals
Case–control	Case–reference	Individuals
Cohort	Follow-up	Individuals
Experimental studies	*Intervention studies*	
Randomized controlled trials	Clinical trials	Patients
Field trials		Healthy people
Community trials	Community intervention studies	Communities

Observational studies allow nature to take its course: the investigator measures but does not intervene. They include studies that can be called descriptive or analytical. A descriptive study is limited to a description of the occurrence of a disease in a population and is often the first step in an epidemiological investigation. An analytical study goes further by analysing relationships between health status and other variables. Apart from the simplest descriptive studies, epidemiological studies are analytical in character.

Limited descriptive information, such as a case series, in which the characteristics of a number of patients with a specific disease are described but are not compared with those of a reference population, often stimulates the initiation of a more detailed epidemiological study. For example, Gottlieb et al. (1981) described four young men with a previously rare form of pneumonia and opened the way for a wide range of epidemiological studies on the condition that became known as AIDS.

Experimental or intervention studies involve an active attempt to change a disease determinant, such as an exposure or a behaviour, or the progress of a disease, through treatment, and are similar in design to experiments in other sciences. However, they are subject to extra constraints, since the health of the people in the study group may be at stake. The major experimental study design is the randomized controlled trial using patients as subjects. Field trials and community trials are other experimental designs, in which the participants are, respectively, healthy people and communities.

In all epidemiological studies it is essential to have a clear definition of a case of the disease being investigated, i.e. the symptoms, signs or other characteristics indicating that a person has the disease. Also necessary is a clear definition of an exposed person, i.e. the characteristics that identify a person as being exposed to the factor under study. In the absence of clear definitions of disease and exposure, great difficulties are likely to be experienced in interpreting the data from an epidemiological study.

Observational epidemiology

Descriptive studies

A simple description of the health status of a community, based on routinely available data or on data obtained in special surveys as described in Chapter 2, is often the first step in an epidemiological investigation. In many countries this type of study is undertaken by a national centre for health statistics. Descriptive studies make no attempt to analyse the links between exposure and effect. They are usually based on death statistics and may examine patterns of death by age, sex or ethnicity during specified time periods or in various countries.

An example of descriptive data is shown in Fig. 3.1, which charts the pattern of maternal mortality in Sweden since the middle of the eighteenth century. The diagram shows the crude maternal death rates per 100 000 live births. The data can be of great value in the identification of factors that have brought about the downward trend. It is interesting to speculate on the possible changes in the living conditions of young women in the 1860s and 1870s which might have caused the temporary rise in maternal mortality at that time.

Fig. 3.2 is also based on routine death statistics and provides an example of the change in death rates over time in three countries. It shows that death rates from stroke have been declining in two of the countries for several decades but increasing in Bulgaria. The next step in the investigation would require information about the comparability of the death certificate records, changes in the incidence and case-fatality of the disease, and changes in risk factors in the populations.

Table 3.2 shows the results of descriptive studies of smoking patterns in certain Pacific islands. It is commonly thought that people in urban areas of developing countries smoke more than rural people but these surveys show the opposite to be true in Fiji and Western Samoa.

Fig. 3.1. Maternal mortality rates in Sweden, 1750–1975

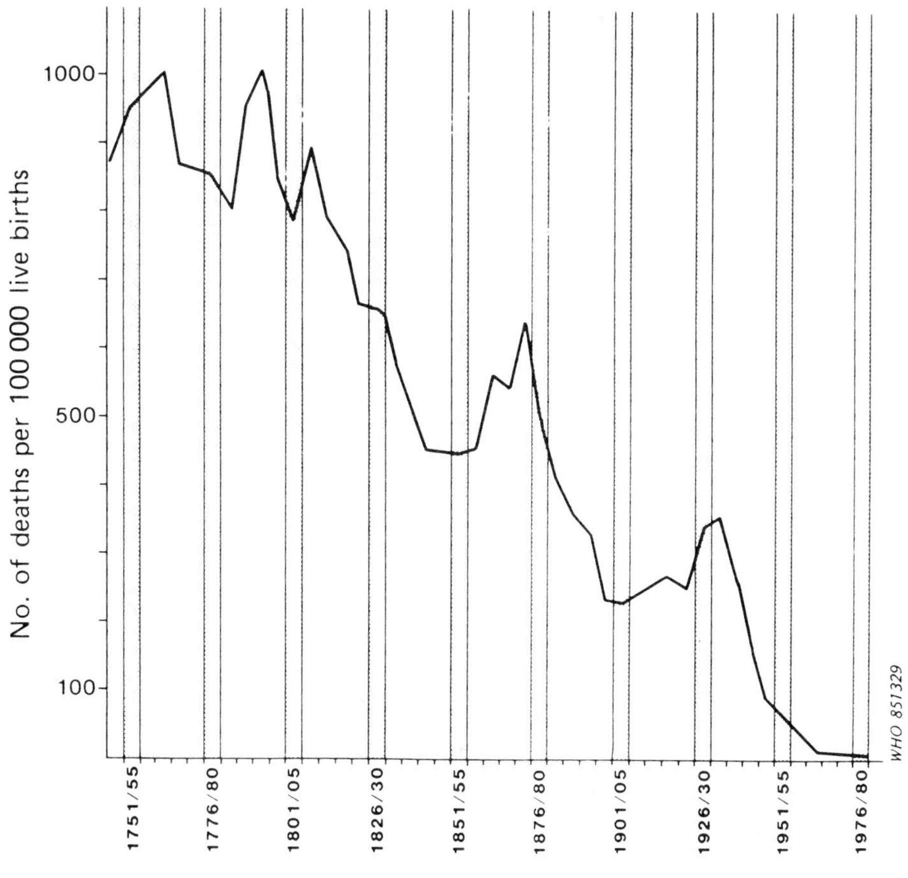

Source: Högberg & Wall, 1986.

Table 3.3 presents results from a descriptive study of serological markers of hepatitis in children in central Tunisia and shows that prevalence increases with age. At the age of 7–9 years over 20% have been exposed to the hepatitis B virus.

Ecological studies

Ecological or correlational studies also frequently initiate the epidemiological process. In an ecological study, the units of analysis are populations or groups of people rather than individuals. For example, in one country, a relationship was demonstrated between average sales of an anti-asthma drug and the occurrence of an unusually high number of asthma deaths (Crane et al., 1989). Such relationships may be studied by comparing populations in different countries at the same time or the same population in one country at different times. The latter approach may avoid some of the socioeconomic confounding (see pages 48–50) that is a potential problem in ecological studies.

Although simple to conduct and thus attractive, ecological studies are often difficult to interpret since it is seldom possible to examine directly the various

Fig. 3.2. Age-standardized death rates from stroke among men aged 40–69, three countries, 1970–1985

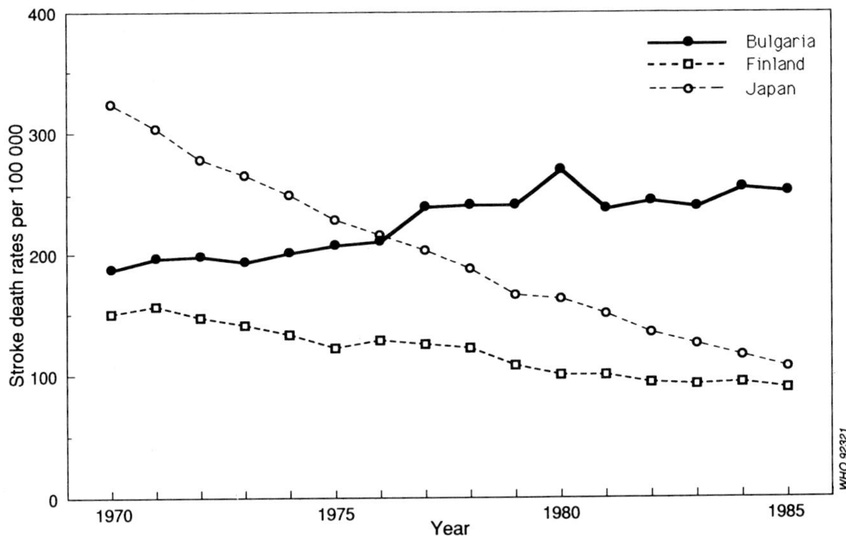

Source: Bonita et al., 1990.

Table 3.2. Prevalence of smoking in adult men in selected Pacific Islands

Country	Percentage of smokers	
	Urban	**Rural**
Fiji		
Melanesian	66	88
Asian Indian	42	62
Kiribati	88	84
New Caledonia	76	41
Western Samoa	57	75

Source: Tuomilehto et al., 1986.

potential explanations for findings. Ecological studies usually rely on data collected for other purposes; data on different exposures and on socioeconomic factors may not be available. In addition, since the unit of analysis is a population or group, the individual link between exposure and effect cannot be made. One attraction of ecological studies is that data can be used from populations with widely differing characteristics. For example, Fig. 3.3 shows oesophageal cancer rates in communities with different patterns of salt consumption; high death rates from oesophageal cancer in certain counties of Henan Province, China, appear to be associated with high salt consumption. It

Table 3.3. Prevalence of hepatitis B markers in blood of children in central Tunisia by age

Age group (years)	Prevalence of hepatitis B markers (%)
1–3	7
4–6	16
7–9	21
10–12	24

Source: Said et al., 1985.

Fig. 3.3. The association between quantity of salt sold and oesophageal cancer mortality in counties of Henan province, China

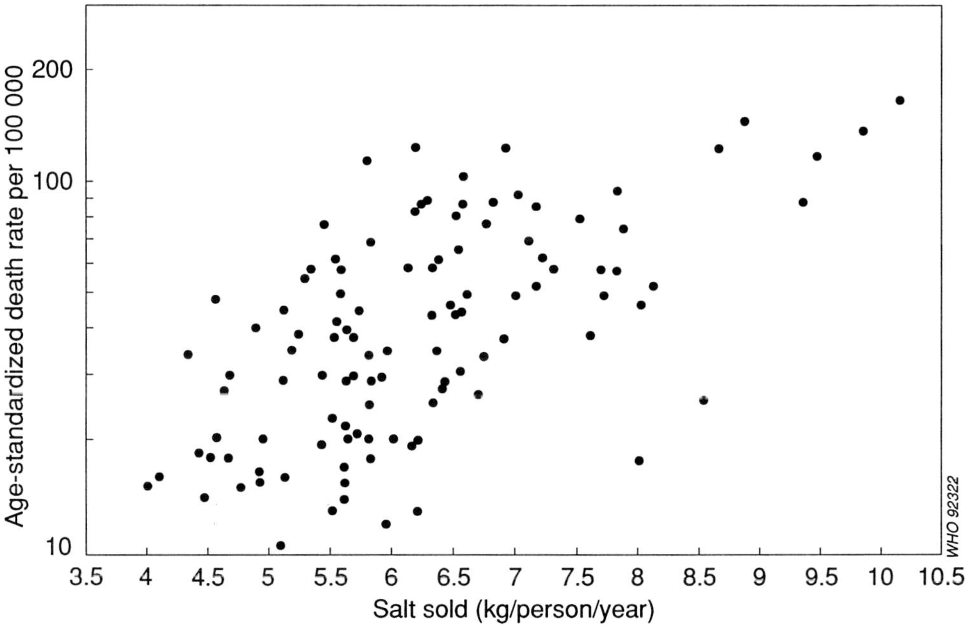

Source: Lu & Qin, 1987. Reproduced by kind permission of the publisher.

is difficult, however, to rule out other possible factors such as an increased consumption of alcohol in areas where there is high salt intake and high rates of oesophageal cancer, alcohol being a known risk factor for this disease.

An ecological fallacy or bias results if inappropriate conclusions are drawn on the basis of ecological data. The association observed between variables at the group level does not necessarily represent the association that exists at the individual level. Ecological studies, however, have often provided a fruitful start for more detailed epidemiological work.

Cross-sectional studies

Cross-sectional studies measure the prevalence of disease and are often called prevalence studies. In a cross-sectional study the measurements of exposure and effect are made at the same time. It is not easy to assess the reasons for associations demonstrated in cross-sectional studies. The key question to be asked is whether the exposure precedes or follows the effect. If the exposure data are known to represent exposure before any effect occurred, the data analysis can be approached in a similar way to that used in cohort studies.

Cross-sectional studies are relatively easy and economical to conduct and are useful for investigating exposures that are fixed characteristics of individuals, such as ethnicity, socioeconomic status, and blood group. In sudden outbreaks of disease a cross-sectional study involving measurement of several exposures is often the most convenient first step in an investigation into the cause.

Several countries conduct regular cross-sectional surveys on representative samples of their populations focusing on personal and demographic characteristics, illnesses and health-related habits. The frequencies of illnesses and other characteristics are then examined in relation to age, sex and ethnicity. Data from cross-sectional studies are helpful in assessing the health care needs of populations.

Cross-sectional surveys of morbidity and the utilization of health services in different countries often give widely varying results, usually reflecting variations in survey methods as well as true differences between populations. Comparisons of morbidity and utilization rates can be hindered by the absence of standardization in survey methods. Recommendations have been made for improving the methodology of health interview surveys in developing countries (Ross & Vaughan, 1986). Attention must be given to the purposes of surveys; questionnaires must be well designed and the sample chosen must be appropriate.

Case–control studies

Case–control studies are relatively simple and economical to carry out and are increasingly used to investigate causes of diseases, especially rare diseases. They include people with a disease (or other outcome variable) of interest and a suitable control group (comparison or reference group) of people unaffected by the disease or outcome variable. The occurrence of the possible cause is compared between cases and controls. Data concerning more than one point in time are collected. Case–control studies are thus longitudinal, in contrast to cross-sectional studies. Case–control studies have been called retrospective studies since the investigator is looking backwards from the disease to a possible cause. This can be confusing because the terms retrospective and prospective are increasingly being used to describe the timing of data collection in relation to the current date. In this sense a case–control study may be either retrospective, when all the data deal with the past, or prospective in which data collection continues with the passage of time.

A case–control study begins with the selection of cases, which should represent all the cases from a specified population (Fig. 3.4). The most difficult task is to

Fig. 3.4. Design of a case-control study

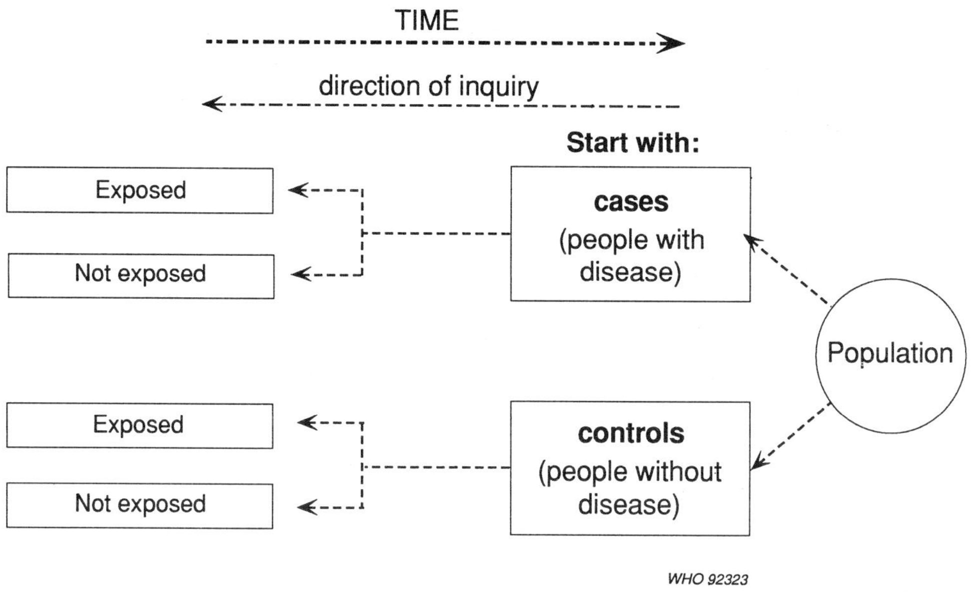

select controls so as to sample the exposure prevalence in the population that generated the cases. Furthermore, the choice of controls and cases must not be influenced by exposure status, which should be determined in the same manner for both. It is not necessary for cases and controls to be all-inclusive; in fact they can be restricted to any specified subgroup, such as old people, males or females.

The controls should represent people who would have been designated study cases if they had developed the disease. Ideally, case–control studies use new (incident) cases to avoid the difficulty of disentangling factors related to causation and survival, although studies have often been conducted using prevalence data (for example, case–control studies of congenital malformations).

An important aspect of case–control studies is the determination of the start and duration of exposure for cases and controls. In the case–control design, the exposure status of the cases is usually determined after the development of the disease (retrospective data) and usually by direct questioning of the affected person or a relative or friend. The informant's answers may be influenced by knowledge about the hypothesis under investigation or the disease experience itself. Exposure is sometimes determined by biochemical measurements (e.g. lead in blood or cadmium in urine), which can be affected by the disease. This problem can be avoided if accurate exposure data are available from an established recording system (e.g. employment records in industry) or if the case–control study is carried out prospectively so that exposure data are collected before the development of the disease. One design of this type is the *nested case–control study* (see pages 40–41).

A classic example of a case–control study was the discovery of the relation between thalidomide and unusual limb defects in babies born in the Federal Republic of Germany in 1959 and 1960; the study, undertaken in 1961, compared affected children with normal children (Mellin & Katzenstein, 1962). Of 46 mothers whose babies had typical malformations, 41 had taken thalidomide between the fourth and ninth weeks of pregnancy, whereas none of the 300 control mothers, whose children were normal, had taken the drug at these stages.

Another example of the use of a case–control study design is shown in Table 3.4. The history of meat consumption was investigated in Papua New Guinea in people with enteritis necroticans, and a comparison was made with people who did not have the disease. Consumption of meat was more likely in the people with disease (50 of 61 cases) than in those who did not have the disease (16 of 57).

Table 3.4. Association between recent meat consumption and enteritis necroticans in Papua New Guinea

		Exposure (recent meat ingestion)		
		Yes	**No**	**Total**
Disease (enteritis necroticans)	**Yes**	50	11	61
	No	16	41	57
	Total	66	52	118

Source: Millar et al., 1985. Reproduced by kind permission of the publisher.

The association of an exposure and a disease is measured in a case–control study by calculation of the odds ratio (OR), which is the ratio of the odds of exposure among the cases to the odds in favour of exposure among the controls. For the data in Table 3.4, the odds ratio is given by:

$$(50/11) \div (16/41)$$

$$= \frac{50 \times 41}{11 \times 16} = 11.6$$

This indicates that the cases were 11.6 times more likely than the controls to have recently ingested meat.

The odds ratio is very similar to the risk ratio (pages 29–30), particularly if a disease is rare.

Cohort studies

Cohort studies, also called follow-up or incidence studies, begin with a group of people (a cohort) free of disease, who are classified into subgroups according to exposure to a potential cause of disease or outcome (Fig. 3.5). Variables of interest are specified and measured and the whole cohort is followed up to see how the subsequent development of new cases of the disease (or other outcome) differs between the groups with and without exposure. Because the data collected refer to different points in time, cohort studies are longitudinal, like case–control studies.

Fig. 3.5. Design of a cohort study

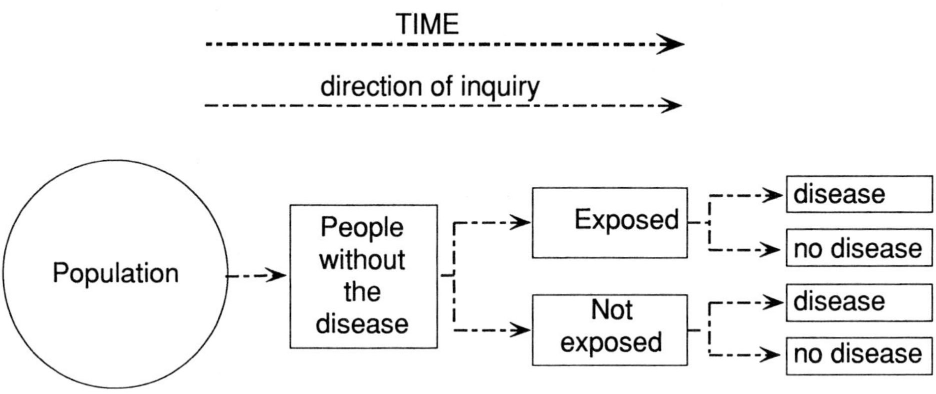

WHO 92324

Cohort studies have been called prospective studies, but this terminology is confusing and should be avoided. As mentioned on page 36, the term "prospective" refers to the timing of data collection and not to the relationship between exposure and effect. Thus there can be both prospective and retrospective cohort studies.

Cohort studies provide the best information about the causation of disease and the most direct measurement of the risk of developing disease. Although conceptually simple, cohort studies are major undertakings and may require long periods of follow-up since disease may occur a long time after exposure. For example, the induction period for leukaemia caused by radiation (i.e. the time required for the specific cause to produce an outcome) is many years and it is necessary to follow up study participants for a correspondingly long time. Many exposures investigated are long-term in nature and accurate information about them requires data collection over long periods. However, in the case of, for example, cigarette smoking, many people have stable habits and information about past exposure can be collected at the time the cohort is defined.

In situations with sudden acute exposures, the cause–effect relationship for acute effects may be obvious, but cohort studies are also used to investigate late or chronic effects. One example is the catastrophic poisoning of residents around a pesticide factory in Bhopal, India, in 1984. An intermediate chemical in the production process, methylisocyanate, leaked from a tank and the fumes drifted into surrounding residential areas, killing more than 2000 people and poisoning 200 000 others. The acute effects were easily studied with a cross-sectional design. More subtle chronic effects and effects developing only after a long latency period are still being studied using cohort study designs.

As cohort studies start with exposed and unexposed people, the difficulties of measuring exposure or finding existing data on individual exposures are important in determining the ease with which this type of study can be carried out. If the disease is rare in the exposed group as well as the unexposed group there may also be problems in ensuring a large enough study group.

The expense of a cohort study can be contained by using routine sources of information about mortality or morbidity, such as disease registers or national registers of deaths as part of the follow-up procedures. Fig. 3.6 presents data from a population-based cohort study of 5914 children in southern Brazil and shows the infant mortality rates for different birth weights. Death during the first year of life is most common for the lightest babies and least common for the heaviest babies. Ideally in cohort studies all subjects would be traced directly, but this may not always be straightforward. In the Brazilian study the proportions of children located at follow-up were reduced in the highest and lowest income groups because of the mobility of these people.

Fig. 3.6. Infant mortality rates according to birth weight in southern Brazil

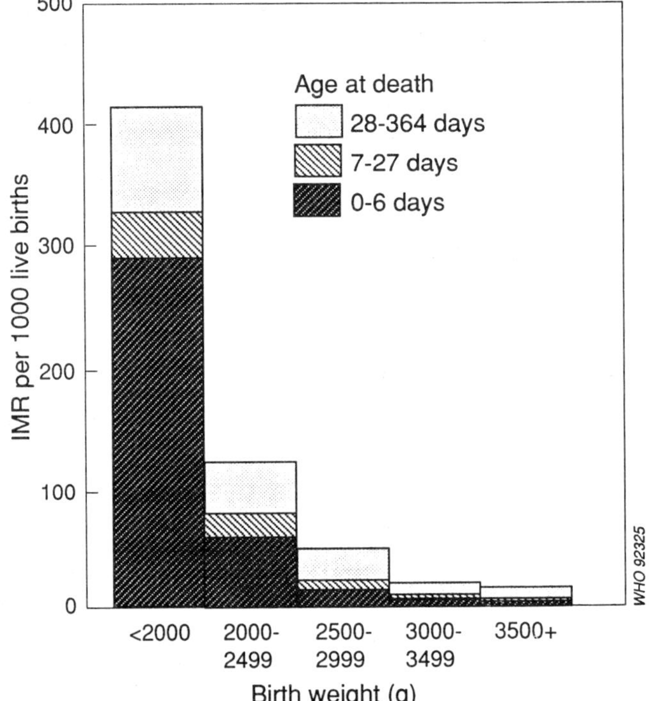

Source: Victora et al., 1987. Reproduced by kind permission of the publisher.

Costs can occasionally be reduced by using a historical cohort (identified on the basis of records of previous exposure). For example, records of exposure of members of the armed services to radioactive fall-out at nuclear bomb testing sites are now being used to examine the possible causal role of fall-out in the development of cancer over the past 30 years. This type of investigation is called a retrospective or historical cohort study, because all the exposure and effect (disease) data have been collected before the actual study begins. This sort of design is relatively common for occupational cancer studies.

The nested case–control design also allows the cost of an epidemiological study to be reduced. The cases and controls are both chosen from a defined cohort, for which some information on exposures and risk factors is already available. Detailed additional information is collected and analysed on the new cases and controls selected for study. This design is particularly useful when measurement of the details of exposure is expensive.

Since cohort studies take healthy people as their starting-point, it is possible to examine a range of outcomes (in contrast to what can be achieved in case–control studies). For example, the Framingham study, a cohort study that began in 1948, has investigated the risk factors not only for cardiovascular diseases but also for a wide range of other diseases, among them respiratory diseases and musculoskeletal disorders.

Although cost remains a major limitation on large cohort studies, methods have been developed to conduct them relatively cheaply. In the study on which Table 2.3 is based, information is collected regularly from a large number of nurses using mailed self-administered questionnaires. Methods are tested on small subsamples, and routine information sources are used to obtain data on disease outcomes. Among many other issues, the relationship between smoking and the risk of stroke in women has been examined. Although stroke is a relatively common cause of death, it is still a rare occurrence in younger women; and so a large cohort is necessary to study its causes.

Tables 3.5 and 3.6 summarize the applications, advantages and disadvantages of the major types of observational study.

Experimental epidemiology

Intervention or experimentation involves attempting to change a variable in one or more groups of people. This could mean the elimination of a dietary factor thought to cause allergy, or testing a new treatment on a selected group of patients. The effects of an intervention are measured by comparing the outcome

Table 3.5. Applications of different observational study designs[a]

	Ecological	Cross-sectional	Case–control	Cohort
Investigation of rare disease	++++	–	+++++	–
Investigation of rare cause	++	–	–	+++++
Testing multiple effects of cause	+	++	–	+++++
Study of multiple exposures and determinants	++	++	++++	+++
Measurements of time relationship	++	–	+[b]	+++++
Direct measurement of incidence	–	–	+[c]	+++++
Investigation of long latent periods	–	–	+++	–

[a] Key: + ... +++++ indicates the degree of suitability
– not suitable

[b] If prospective.

[c] If population-based.

Table 3.6. Advantages and disadvantages of different observational study designs

	Ecological	Cross-sectional	Case–control	Cohort
Probability of:				
selection bias	NA	medium	high	low
recall bias	NA	high	high	low
loss to follow-up	NA	NA	low	high
confounding	high	medium	medium	low
Time required	low	medium	medium	high
Cost	low	medium	medium	high

NA: not applicable.

in the experimental group with that in a control group. Since the interventions are strictly determined by the protocol, ethical considerations are of paramount importance in the design of these studies. For example, no patient should be denied appropriate treatment as a result of participation in an experiment, and the treatment being tested must be acceptable in the light of current knowledge.

This type of study can take one of three forms:

- randomized controlled trial;
- field trial;
- community trial.

Randomized controlled trials

A randomized controlled trial (or randomized clinical trial) is an epidemiological experiment to study a new preventive or therapeutic regimen. Subjects in a population are randomly allocated to groups, usually called treatment and control groups, and the results are assessed by comparing the outcome in the two or more groups. The outcome of interest will vary but may be the development of new disease or recovery from established disease.

The design of a randomized controlled trial is shown in Fig. 3.7. To ensure that the groups being compared are equivalent, patients are allocated to them randomly, i.e. by chance. Within the limits of chance, randomization ensures that control and treatment groups will be comparable at the start of an investigation; any differences between groups are chance occurrences unaffected by the conscious or unconscious biases of the investigators.

The intervention under test may be a new drug or a new regimen, such as early mobilization after myocardial infarction. All subjects in the trial must meet the specified criteria for the condition under investigation, and other criteria are usually specified to ensure a reasonably homogeneous group of subjects, e.g. only patients with long-standing or mild disease. The details of a randomized controlled trial of early discharge from hospital after myocardial infarction are shown in Fig. 3.8. The study suggests that, for carefully selected patients with uncomplicated myocardial infarction, discharge after three days does not harm

Fig. 3.7. Design of a randomized controlled trial

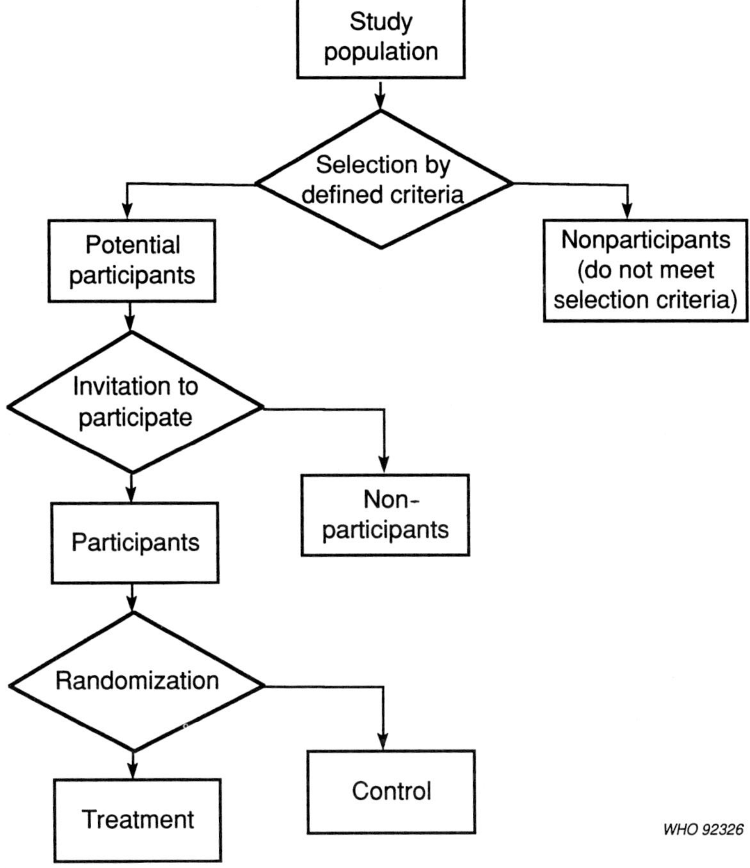

the patient. Fewer were readmitted or had subsequent problems than in the late-discharge group. However, only a small proportion of all myocardial infarction patients were included in the study, and its power was thus limited because of the small sample size (see page 46).

Randomized controlled trials have been helpful in assessing the value of new therapies to combat acute diseases in developing countries. For example, a trial using rice-based or glucose-based oral rehydration solution involved 342 patients with acute watery diarrhoea during an epidemic of cholera in Bangladesh in 1983 (Molla et al., 1985). The patients were randomly assigned to treatment with either glucose-based or rice-based oral rehydration solution. The study showed that the glucose component of oral rehydration solution could be replaced by rice powder with improved results, as indicated by decreases in mean stool output and intake of solution. Studies such as this have important implications for the efficient use of health-care resources in developing countries. Glucose is a costly manufactured product and is not always available in countries where diarrhoeal diseases are a major problem.

Fig. 3.8. Randomized controlled trial of early hospital discharge after myocardial infarction

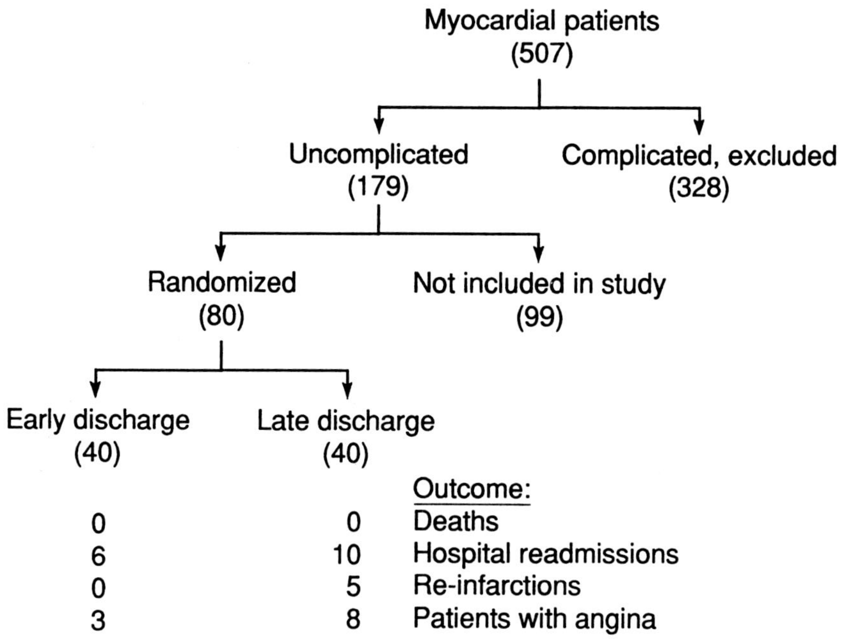

Myocardial patients
(507)

Uncomplicated
(179)

Complicated, excluded
(328)

Randomized
(80)

Not included in study
(99)

Early discharge (40)	Late discharge (40)	Outcome:
0	0	Deaths
6	10	Hospital readmissions
0	5	Re-infarctions
3	8	Patients with angina

WHO 92327

Source: Topol et al., 1988. Reproduced by kind permission of the publisher.

Field trials

Field trials, in contrast to clinical trials, involve people who are disease-free but presumed to be at risk; data collection takes place "in the field", usually among non-institutionalized people in the general population. Since the subjects are disease-free and the purpose is to prevent the occurrence of diseases that may occur with relatively low frequency, field trials are often huge undertakings involving major logistic and financial considerations. For example, one of the largest field trials ever undertaken was that of the Salk vaccine for the prevention of poliomyelitis, which involved over one million children. Even the study of the prevention of coronary heart disease in high-risk middle-aged males involved screening 360 000 men to identify 12 866 people eligible for the trial. In each of these two examples, randomization was used to allocate participants to various treatment groups.

A field trial of a new vaccine against New World cutaneous leishmaniasis was conducted in Brazil (Fig. 3.9). Brazilian army recruits with relatively high rates of infection were used to test the efficacy of the vaccine against a placebo. The vaccine produced a high rate of skin conversion, indicating that antibodies had been generated. However, the same proportion of each group developed the disease, suggesting that the vaccine was not effective, although the incidence of the disease was perhaps too low to permit satisfactory evaluation.

Fig. 3.9. Field trial of vaccine against New World cutaneous leishmaniasis (NWCL)

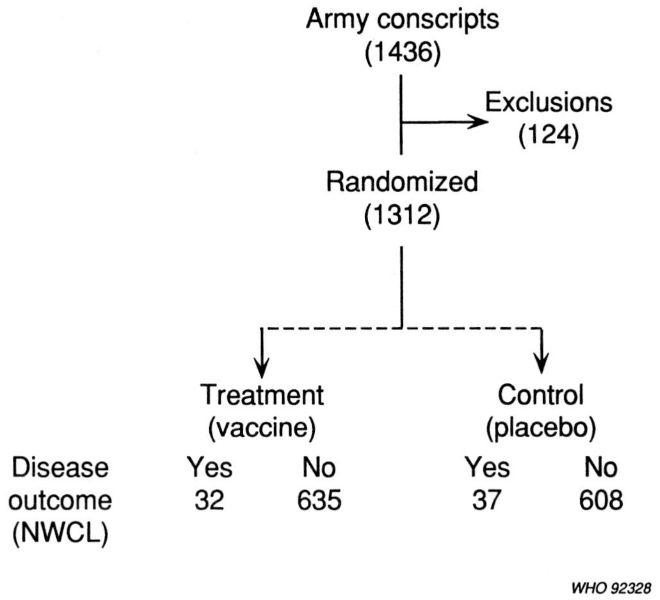

Source: Antunes et al., 1986. Reproduced by kind permission of the publisher.

The field trial method can be used to evaluate interventions aimed at reducing exposure without necessarily measuring the occurrence of health effects. For instance, different protective methods for pesticide exposure have been tested in this way and measurement of blood lead levels in children has shown the protection provided by elimination of lead paint in the home environment. Such intervention studies can often be carried out on a small scale at low cost.

Community trials

In this form of experiment the treatment groups are communities rather than individuals. This is particularly appropriate for diseases that have their origins in social conditions, which in turn can most easily be influenced by intervention directed at group behaviour as well as at individuals. Cardiovascular disease is a good example of a condition appropriate for community trials (Farquhar et al., 1977), several of which are under way in this field (Salonen et al., 1986). A limitation of such studies is that only a small number of communities can be included and random allocation of communities is not practicable; other methods are required to ensure that any differences found at the end of the study can be attributed to the intervention rather than to inherent differences between communities. Furthermore, it is difficult to isolate the communities where intervention is taking place from general social changes that may be occurring. Consequently this type of study may underestimate the effect of intervention.

Potential errors in epidemiological studies

An important purpose of most epidemiological investigations is to measure accurately the occurrence of disease (or other outcome). Epidemiological measurement is, however, not easy and there are many possibilities for errors in measurement. Much attention is devoted to minimizing errors and, since they can never be eliminated, assessing their importance. Error can be either random or systematic.

Random error

Random error is the divergence, due to chance alone, of an observation on a sample from the true population value, leading to lack of precision in the measurement of an association. There are three major sources of random error: individual biological variation, sampling error, and measurement error.

Random error can never be completely eliminated since we can study only a sample of the population, individual variation always occurs and no measurement is perfectly accurate. Random error can be reduced by the careful measurement of exposure and outcome thus making individual measurements as precise as possible. Sampling error occurs as part of the process of selecting study participants who are always a sample of a larger population, and the best way to reduce it is to increase the size of the study.

Sample size calculations

The desirable size of a proposed study can be assessed using standard formulae. Information on the following variables is required before the formulae can be employed:

- required level of statistical significance of the expected result;
- acceptable chance of missing a real effect;
- magnitude of the effect under investigation;
- amount of disease in the population;
- relative sizes of the groups being compared.

In reality, sample size is often determined by logistic and financial considerations, and a compromise always has to be made between sample size and costs. A practical guide to determining sample size in health studies has been published by WHO (Lwanga & Lemeshow, 1991).

The precision of a study can also be improved by ensuring that the groups are of appropriate relative size. This is often an issue of concern in case–control studies when a decision is required on the number of controls to be chosen for each case. It is not possible to be definitive about the ideal ratio of controls to cases, since this depends on the relative costs of accumulating cases and controls. If cases are scarce and controls plentiful, it is appropriate to increase the ratio of controls to cases. For example, in the case–control study of the effects of thalidomide (pages 37–38), 46 affected children were compared with 300 normal children. In general, however, there may be little point in having more than four controls for each case. It is important to ensure that there is sufficient similarity between cases and controls when the data are to be analysed by, for example, age group or social class; if most cases and only a few controls were in the older age groups, the study would be inefficient and much time and effort wasted.

Systematic error

Systematic error (or bias) occurs in epidemiology when there is a tendency to produce results that differ in a systematic manner from the true values. A study with a small systematic error is said to have a high accuracy. Accuracy is not affected by sample size.

Systematic error is a particular hazard because epidemiologists usually have no control over participants in studies unlike the situation in laboratory experiments. Furthermore, it is often difficult to obtain representative samples of source populations. Some variables of interest in epidemiology are particularly difficult to measure, among them personality type, alcohol consumption habits, and past exposures to rapidly changing environmental conditions, and this difficulty may lead to systematic error.

The possible sources of systematic error in epidemiology are many and varied; over 30 specific types of bias have been identified. The principal biases are:

- selection bias;
- measurement (or classification) bias.

Confounding, which provides misleading estimates of effect, is not strictly a type of bias, since it does not result from systematic error in research design. It arises because non-random distribution of risk factors in the source population also occurs in the study population.

Selection bias

Selection bias occurs when there is a systematic difference between the characteristics of the people selected for a study and the characteristics of those who are not. An obvious source of selection bias occurs when participants select themselves for a study, either because they are unwell or because they are particularly worried about an exposure. It is well known, for example, that people who respond to an invitation to participate in a study on the effects of smoking differ in their smoking habits from non-responders; the latter are usually heavier smokers. In studies of children's health, where parental cooperation is required, selection bias may also occur. In a cohort study of newborn children (Victora et al., 1987), the proportion successfully followed up for 12 months varied according to income level of the parents. If individuals entering or remaining in a study display different associations from those who do not, a biased estimate of the association between exposure and outcome is produced.

An important selection bias is introduced when the disease or factor under investigation itself makes people unavailable for study. For example, in a factory where workers are exposed to formaldehyde, those who suffer most from eye irritation are likely to leave their jobs at their own request or after medical advice. The remaining workers are less affected and a prevalence study in the workplace of the association between formaldehyde exposure and eye irritation may be very misleading.

In occupational epidemiology studies there is, by definition, a very important selection bias called the healthy worker effect (Chapter 9): workers have to be healthy enough to perform their duties; the severely ill and disabled are ordinarily excluded from employment. Similarly, if a study is based on examinations carried out in a health centre and there is no follow-up of participants who do not return, biased results may be produced: unwell patients may be in bed either at home or in hospital. All epidemiological study designs need to take this type of selection bias into account.

Measurement bias

Measurement bias occurs when the individual measurements or classifications of disease or exposure are inaccurate (i.e. they do not measure correctly what they are supposed to measure). There are many sources of measurement bias and their effects are of varying importance. For instance, biochemical or physiological measurements are never completely accurate and different laboratories often produce different results on the same specimen. If the specimens of the exposed and control groups are analysed randomly by different laboratories with insufficient joint quality assurance procedures, the errors will be random and less potentially serious for the epidemiological analysis than in the situation where all specimens from the exposed group are analysed in one laboratory and all those from the control group are analysed in another. If the laboratories produce systematically different results when analysing the same specimen, the epidemiological evaluation becomes biased.

A form of measurement bias of particular importance in retrospective case–control studies is known as recall bias. This occurs when there is a differential recall of information by cases and controls; for instance, cases may be more likely to recall past exposure, especially if it is widely known to be associated with the disease under study (for example, lack of exercise and heart disease). Recall bias can either exaggerate the degree of effect associated with the exposure (as with heart patients being more likely to admit to a past lack of exercise) or underestimate it (if cases are more likely than controls to deny past exposure).

If measurement bias occurs equally in the groups being compared (non-differential bias) it almost always results in an underestimate of the true strength of the relationship. This form of bias may account for some apparent discrepancies between the results of different epidemiological studies.

Confounding

In a study of the association between exposure to a cause (or risk factor) and the occurrence of disease, confounding can occur when another exposure exists in the study population and is associated both with the disease and the exposure being studied. A problem arises if this extraneous factor—itself a determinant or risk factor for the health outcome—is unequally distributed between the exposure subgroups. Confounding occurs when the effects of two exposures (risk factors) have not been separated and it is therefore incorrectly concluded that the effect is due to one rather than the other variable. For instance, in a study of the association between tobacco smoking and lung cancer, age would be a confounding factor if the average ages of the nonsmoking and smoking groups in the study population were very different since lung cancer incidence increases with age.

Confounding can have a very important influence, possibly even changing the apparent direction of an association. A variable that appears to be protective may, after control of confounding, be found to be harmful. The most common concern over confounding is that it may create the appearance of a cause–effect relationship that in reality does not exist. For a variable to be a confounder, it must, in its own right, be a determinant of the occurrence of disease (i.e. a risk factor) and with the exposure under investigation. Thus, in a study of radon exposure and lung cancer, smoking is not a confounder if the smoking habits are identical in the radon-exposed and control groups.

Age and social class are often confounders in epidemiological studies. An association between high blood pressure and coronary heart disease may in truth represent concomitant changes in the two variables that occur with increasing age; the potential confounding effect of age has to be considered, and when this is done it is seen that high blood pressure indeed increases the risk of coronary heart disease.

Another example of confounding is shown in Fig. 3.10. Confounding may be the explanation for the relationship demonstrated between coffee consumption and the risk of coronary heart disease, since it is known that coffee consumption is associated with cigarette smoking: people who drink coffee are more likely to smoke than people who do not drink coffee. It is also well known that cigarette smoking is a cause of coronary heart disease. It is thus possible that the relationship between coffee consumption and coronary heart disease merely

Fig. 3.10. Confounding: coffee drinking, cigarette smoking, and coronary heart disease

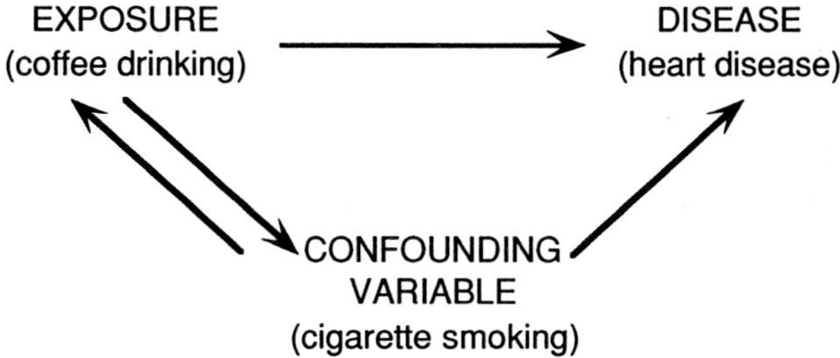

WHO 92329

reflects the known causal association of smoking with the disease. In this situation, smoking confounds the apparent relationship between coffee consumption and coronary heart disease.

The control of confounding

Several methods are available to control confounding, either through study design or during the analysis of results.

The methods commonly used to control confounding in the design of an epidemiological study are:

- randomization;
- restriction;
- matching.

At the analysis stage, confounding can be controlled by:

- stratification;
- statistical modelling.

Randomization, which is applicable only to experimental studies, is the ideal method for ensuring that potential confounding variables are equally distributed among the groups being compared. The sample sizes have to be sufficiently large to avoid random maldistribution of such variables. Randomization avoids the association between potentially confounding variables and the exposure that is being considered.

Restriction can be used to limit the study to people who have particular characteristics. For example, in a study on the effects of coffee on coronary heart disease, participation in the study could be restricted to nonsmokers, thus removing any potential effect of confounding by cigarette smoking.

If *matching* is used to control confounding the study participants are selected so as to ensure that potential confounding variables are evenly distributed in the two groups being compared. For example, in a case–control study of exercise and coronary heart disease, each patient with heart disease can be matched with a control of the same age group and sex to ensure that confounding by age and sex does not occur. Matching has been used extensively in case–control studies but it can lead to problems in the selection of controls if the matching criteria are too strict or too numerous; this is called overmatching.

Matching can be expensive and time-consuming, but is particularly useful if the danger exists of there being no overlap between cases and controls, as where the cases are likely to be older than the controls.

In large studies it is usually preferable to control for confounding in the analytical phase rather than in the design phase. Confounding can then be controlled by *stratification*, which involves the measurement of the strength of associations in well-defined and homogeneous categories (strata) of the confounding variable. If age is a confounder, the association may be measured in, say, 10-year age groups; if sex or ethnicity is a confounder, the association is measured separately in men and women or in the different ethnic groups. Methods are available for summarizing the overall association by producing a weighted average of the estimates calculated in each separate stratum.

Although stratification is conceptually simple and relatively easy to carry out, it is often limited by the size of the study and it cannot help to control many factors simultaneously, as is often necessary. In this situation, statistical *modelling* (multivariate) is required to estimate the strength of the associations while controlling for a number of confounding variables simultaneously; a range of statistical techniques is available for these analyses (Dixon & Massey, 1969).

Validity

Validity is an expression of the degree to which a test is capable of measuring what it is intended to measure. A study is valid if its results correspond to the truth; there should be no systematic error (page 47) and the random error should be as small as possible. Fig. 3.11 indicates the relationship between the true value and measured values for low and high validity and reliability. With low reliability but high validity the measured values are spread out, but the mean of the measured values is close to the true value. On the other hand, a high reliability (or repeatability) of the measurements does not ensure validity since they may all be far from the true value. There are two types of validity: internal and external.

Fig. 3.11. Validity and reliability

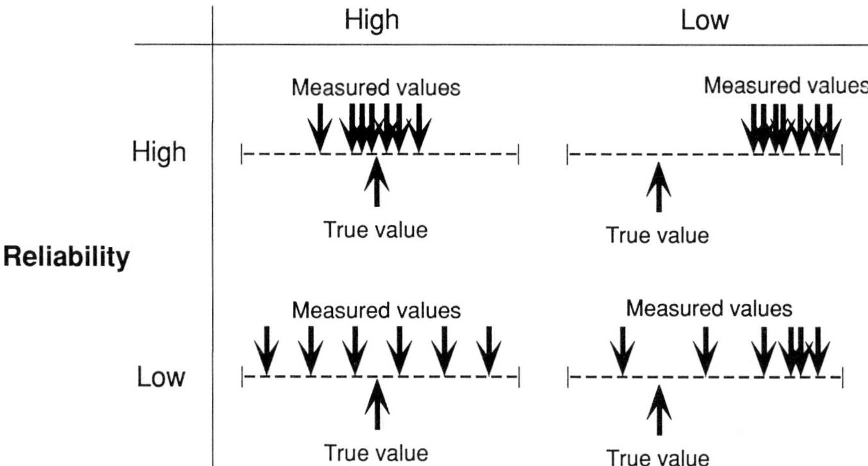

Internal validity

Internal validity is the degree to which the results of an observation are correct for the particular group of people being studied. For example, measurements of blood haemoglobin must distinguish accurately participants with anaemia as defined in the study. Analysis of the blood in a different laboratory may produce different results because of systematic error, but the evaluation of associations with anaemia, as measured by one laboratory, may still be internally valid.

For a study to be of any use it must be internally valid, although even a study that is perfectly valid internally may be of no consequence because the results cannot be compared with other studies. Internal validity can be threatened by all sources of systematic error but can be improved by good design and attention to detail.

External validity

External validity or generalizability is the extent to which the results of a study apply to people not in it (or, for example, to laboratories not involved in it). Internal validity is necessary for, but does not guarantee, external validity, and is easier to achieve. External validity requires external quality control of the measurements and judgements about the degree to which the results of a study can be extrapolated. This does not require that the study sample be representative of a reference population. For example, evidence that the effect of lowering blood cholesterol in men is also relevant to women requires a judgement about the external validity of studies in men. External validity is assisted by study designs that examine clearly-stated hypotheses in well-defined populations.

Ethical issues

Guidelines on the general conduct of biomedical research are contained in the Declaration of Helsinki and *Ethics and epidemiology: international guidelines*, published by the Council for International Organizations of Medical Sciences (Bankowski et al., 1991). The practice of epidemiology requires adherence to the basic principles of biomedical ethics and carries special obligations to individuals and communities, not only those participating in studies but also others whose health may be protected or improved by application of the results. People who have been exposed to a health hazard should realize that epidemiological studies carried out on them may not improve their personal situation but may help to protect thousands of other people.

Free and voluntary informed consent must be obtained from participants in studies and they must retain the right to withdraw at any time. However, it may prove impracticable for informed consent to be given for access to routine medical records. Epidemiologists must respect personal privacy and confidentiality at all times. They have an obligation to tell communities what they are doing and why, and to transmit the results of studies, and their significance, to the communities involved. All proposals for epidemiological studies should be submitted to properly constituted institutional ethics committees before work begins.

Study questions

3.1 What are the applications and disadvantages of the major epidemiological study designs?

3.2 Outline the design of a case–control study and a cohort study to examine the association of a high-fat diet with bowel cancer.

3.3 What is random error and how can it be reduced?

3.4 What are the main types of systematic error in epidemiological studies and how can their effects be reduced?

Chapter 4
Basic statistics

Statistics is the science of summarizing and analysing data that are subject to random variation (Last, 1988). The term is also applied to the data themselves and to summary measures based on them. Clearly, statistics is a very important tool in epidemiology. This chapter gives a brief account of some basic statistical concepts and techniques. Further study will be required by the reader who wishes to plan and carry out an epidemiological study (see, for example, Colton, 1974; Dixon & Massey, 1969; Lwanga & Tye, 1986).

Distributions and summary measures

Distributions

Methods of presenting data depend partly on the type of data collected. There are four broad categories of measurement scale: (1) nominal scales, in which observations are classified into categories (e.g., classification of disease, gender); (2) ordinal scales, which assign rank orders to categories (e.g., mild, moderate, and severe); (3) interval scales, in which the distance between two measurements are defined (e.g., temperature, scores on intelligence tests); and (4) ratio scales, in which both the distance and ratio between two measurements are defined (e.g., length, incidence of disease, number of children). In both ratio and interval scales, it is possible to specify the extent to which one measurement is larger than another (e.g. 70 °C is 35 degrees warmer than 35 °C, one metre is 50 cm longer than 50 cm). However, a ratio scale has the additional possibility of specifying the ratio between two measurements (e.g. one metre is twice as long as 50 cm).

Measurement scales are called *continuous* if they can be continuously refined to measure more accurately. For example, no matter how accurately length is measured, it is always possible to make a more accurate measurement by further subdividing the measurement instrument. Measurements are *discrete* if such refinements are not always possible. For example, it is not possible to refine continuously the measurement of the number of children because there are no possible values between 0 and 1, 1 and 2, and so on.

Data can be presented in various forms, including frequency tables, histograms, bar charts, cross-tabulations and pie charts.

A frequency distribution can often be presented as a table showing the number of times that data with particular characteristics occur in a data set (Lwanga & Tye, 1986). The distribution tells how many or what proportion of the group has each value or range of values out of all possible values (Table 4.1). A frequency table can be used with any type of measurement scale. If necessary, data can be grouped as in Table 4.1.

Table 4.1. Distribution of mercury concentrations in hair of 300 high school students

Mercury concentration (μg/g)	No. of children
0–0.49	95
0.5–0.99	91
1.0–1.49	47
1.5–1.99	30
2.0–2.49	16
2.5–2.99	8
3.0–3.49	9
3.5–3.99	4

Adapted from Kjellström et al., 1982.

A frequency distribution can be represented graphically by a bar chart for discrete data or by a histogram for continuous data. In a bar chart, the frequencies are listed along one axis, usually the vertical, and the categories are listed along the other axis, usually the horizontal. The frequency of each group is represented by the length of the corresponding bar (see Fig. 4.1 for an example of a bar chart). A histogram is similar except that intervals are used in place of categories. Fig. 4.2 is a histogram of the frequency distribution in Table 4.1.

In a histogram the size of the intervals chosen can vary. The smaller the intervals, the more detailed the histogram. As the intervals become smaller and more numerous the shape of the histogram becomes increasingly like a smooth curve. Fig. 4.3 shows a smooth curve, which approximates the distribution presented in Fig. 4.2. Frequency distributions for continuous measures are often presented in the form of a smooth curve.

Fig. 4.1. Bar chart showing prevalence of rheumatoid arthritis among men and women over 55 years of age in the USA and Indonesia

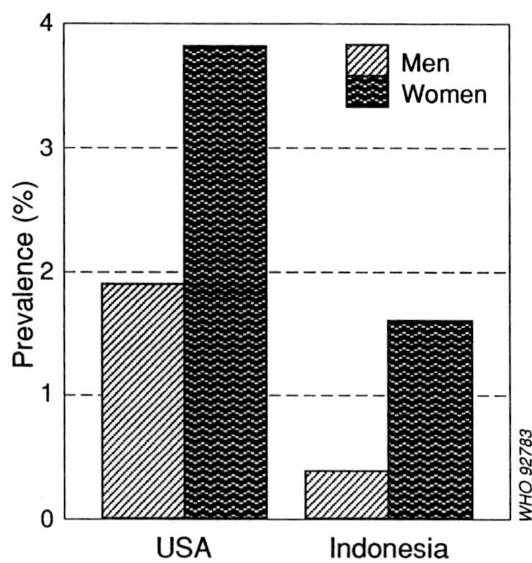

Source: Darmawan, 1988.

Fig. 4.2. Histogram of mercury concentrations in hair of 300 high school students

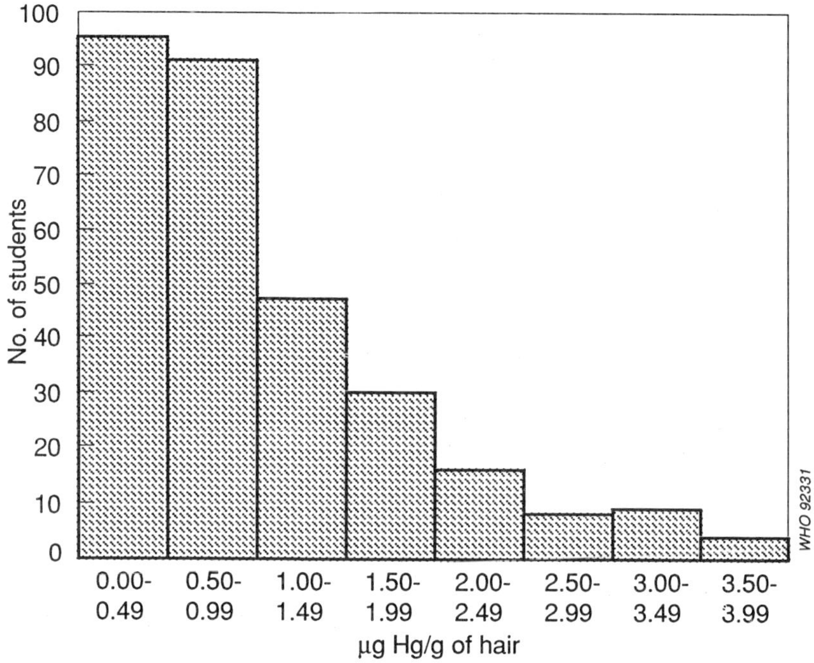

Source: Kjellström et al., 1982. Reproduced by kind permission of the publisher.

Fig. 4.3. Smooth curve fitted to the data shown in Fig. 4.2

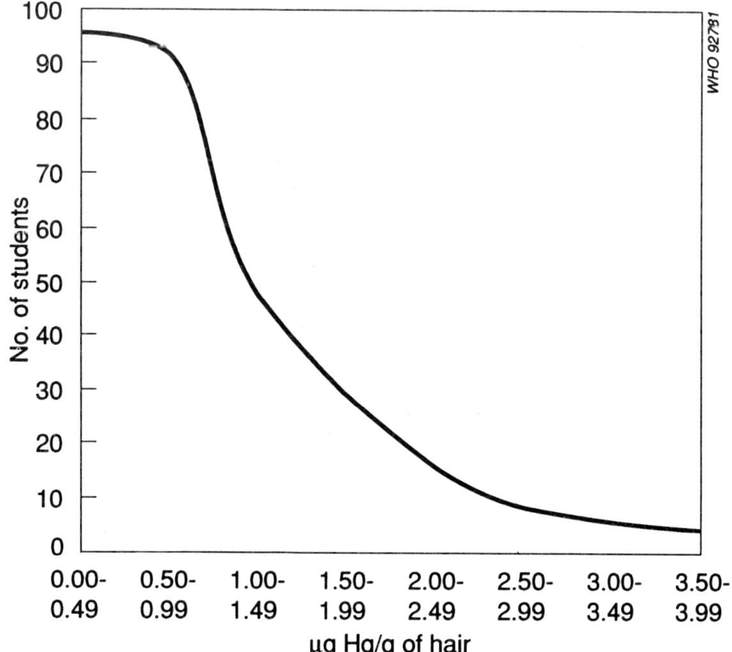

Two basic characteristics that can be used to summarize distributions for interval and ratio scale data are measures of central tendency (also called central location; indicating the middle of the distribution) and measures of variability (indicating the spread of values).

Measures of central tendency

The mean, median and mode are measures of the central tendency of a distribution.

The mean (or average value) is designated $\bar{x}$ and can be calculated from the frequency distribution by summing the values of all the observations (x_i) and dividing by the number of observations (n).

The median value (the middle value) is the value on the scale that divides the distribution into two equal parts. Half of the observations have a value less than or equal to the median, and half have a value greater than or equal to the median. In order to calculate the median of a set of observations, first arrange the observations in order, according to their value on the measurement scale. If n is an odd number, then the median will be the value corresponding to the middle observation. If there are an even number of observations, then the median is the average of the two middle observations. For example, to find the median of the numbers 3, 8, 2, 4, 7, 8, first arrange them in rank order as follows: 2, 3, 4, 7, 8, 8. The median is then the average of the two middle observations, 4 and 7, i.e., 5.5.

The mode is the most frequently occurring value in a set of observations. In the above example the mode is 8.

Measures of variability

Although measures of central tendency are very useful for summarizing a frequency distribution, they do not indicate the spread of values and differently shaped curves may have the same central tendency. It is therefore necessary to provide information on variability, in addition to measures of central tendency, in order to give a clearer idea of the shape of the distribution.

The range, the semiquartile range and the standard deviation are commonly used measures of variability or dispersion. The range indicates the distance between the highest and lowest values. The semiquartile range is based on quantiles, which are divisions of a distribution into equal, ordered subgroups, deciles are tenths; quartiles, quarters; quintiles, fifths; terciles, thirds; and centiles, hundredths. The semiquartile range is the range of the middle two quartiles. Thus, the semiquartile range gives the distance between the upper and lower boundaries of the middle half of the distribution.

The standard deviation is the square root of the variance. To calculate the variance, the squares of the differences of the individual observations from the mean are added together, and the resulting sum of squares is divided by the number of observations minus one. The abbreviations s^2 and s or SD are often used to refer to the variance and standard deviation respectively.

$$\text{Thus} \quad s^2 = \sum_1^n (x_i - \bar{x})^2/(n-1)$$

Normal and log normal distributions

The standard deviation is especially useful when the underlying distribution is approximately normal (Gaussian), i.e. symmetrically bell-shaped (see Fig. 4.4). This is often assumed to be the case for many biological characteristics, among them height, weight and blood pressure.

The normal distribution has extremely useful characteristics. A large number of statistical tests and calculations can be used if the observations follow a normal distribution. In addition, approximately two-thirds of the values under a normal distribution curve fall within one standard deviation of the mean, and approximately 95% fall within two standard deviations of the mean.

The log normal distribution is also commonly used in epidemiology. It is highly skewed but the logarithms of the values are normally distributed. Levels of chemicals in blood of individuals who have been exposed to pollution often have log normal distributions (see Chapter 9). By using the logarithms of measured blood values, data can be analysed using all the features of a normal distribution. The mean of the logarithms can be converted back by anti-log to give the geometric mean of the data. In skewed distributions that are close to log normal, this mean will be close to the median. By converting back the standard deviation of the logarithms, the geometric standard deviation of the measured values is calculated.

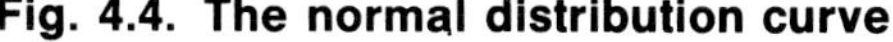

Fig. 4.4. The normal distribution curve

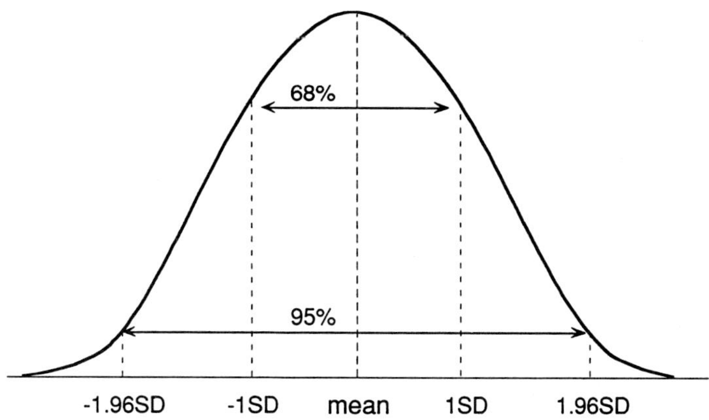

WHO 92332

Estimation

Populations and samples

Usually it is not possible to study the entire population in which one is interested. It is therefore necessary to consider a sample and to relate its characteristics to the total population. Ideally, every individual in the population from which the sample is drawn should have a known chance of being included in the sample. A simple random sample is one in which each individual in the population has an equal chance of being drawn. A common way to select a simple random sample is to use random number tables, which are available in many elementary statistical textbooks (e.g., Dixon & Massey, 1969). The first step is to assign a unique number to each individual in the population. The second step is to choose a starting-point in the random number table (you may begin anywhere in the table). Read the number where you have started. If that number corresponds to a number in your sample, then the corresponding individual should be chosen. Repeat the process with the next number from the random number table, continuing until the requisite number of observations for your sample has been chosen.

The random numbers given in most textbooks are usually six or eight digits long. If your population size is only two or three digits long, as is commonly the case, it would be more efficient to consider only the first few digits of the random numbers.

Some computer programs and some hand-held calculators are able to generate random numbers of any length. These can be used in place of random number tables.

If repeated samples are taken from the same population, the statistical measures of central tendency and variability, such as the mean, median and standard deviation, vary between samples. The degree of variation depends on both the amount of variation in the population and the size of the samples. One of the most important rules of statistics is that, even if the underlying population is not normally distributed, the means of the samples themselves will be approximately normally distributed if the sample sizes are sufficiently large. The standard deviation of the sample means is called the standard error of the mean; it is calculated by dividing the standard deviation of a sample by the square root of the sample size:

$$\mathrm{SE} = s/\sqrt{n}.$$

The standard error of the mean is sometimes incorrectly used to summarize data. Unlike the standard deviation, it does not summarize the variability in the observations or give an insight into their range. The standard error of the mean is always smaller than the standard deviation of the sample.

Confidence intervals

Once the sample has been drawn, it can be used to estimate characteristics of the underlying population. Because estimates vary from sample to sample, it is important to know how close the estimate derived from any one sample is likely to be to the underlying population value. One way to find this out is to construct a confidence interval around the estimate, i.e., to construct a range of values surrounding the estimate which have a specified probability of including the true population values. The specified probability is called the confidence level and the endpoints of the confidence interval are the confidence limits.

To calculate the confidence limits around an estimated population mean it is necessary to have measures of (1) variation such as the population standard deviation σ, (2) the estimated mean ($\bar{x}$), (3) the sample size (n), and (4) the specified probability of including the true population value. If we assume that the underlying population is normally distributed with a known standard deviation σ, then the formula for calculating the limits of a 95% confidence interval around the mean is as follows:

$$\text{lower limit} = \bar{x} - \frac{1.96\sigma}{\sqrt{n}}$$

$$\text{upper limit} = \bar{x} + \frac{1.96\sigma}{\sqrt{n}}$$

(For a 90% confidence interval replace 1.96 by 1.67.)

As an illustration, suppose in a random sample of 100 factory workers, the mean blood lead concentration ($\bar{x}$) was 90 μg/l. Suppose further that the level of concentration of lead in blood is normally distributed with a standard deviation of 10 (i.e., $\sigma = 10$). Then the limits of the 95% confidence interval around the estimate can be calculated as follows:

$$\text{lower limit} = 90 - \frac{1.96 \times 10}{\sqrt{100}} = 88.04$$

$$\text{upper limit} = 90 + \frac{1.96 \times 10}{\sqrt{100}} = 91.96$$

Thus the confidence interval ranges from 88.04 to 91.96.

A sample estimate is usually presented along with its confidence interval. It is important to realize that the size of the confidence interval is related to the size of the sample: the larger the sample, the smaller the confidence interval for a given confidence level. The size of the confidence interval is also related to the confidence level specified. For a given data set, the higher the confidence level specified, the larger is the confidence interval. This can be seen clearly in Fig. 4.5, which presents confidence intervals associated with different confidence levels for the same data.

Statistical inference

Hypothesis testing

Hypothesis testing is a method used by statisticians and epidemiologists to determine how likely it is that observed differences in data are entirely due to

Fig. 4.5. Confidence intervals associated with different confidence levels

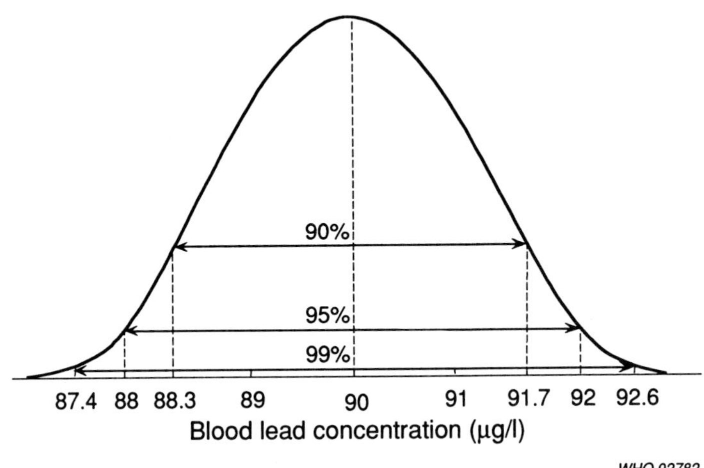

sampling error rather than to underlying population differences. The null hypothesis is useful in this process. It states that any observed differences are entirely due to sampling errors (i.e. to chance).

A statistical formula (based on assumptions about the distribution of the data in the underlying population) is used to calculate the probability that differences at least as large as those found in the observed data would have occurred by chance. This probability is known as the *P*-value. If the *P*-value is low, this indicates that differences at least as large as those observed occur by chance in only a small proportion of all possible samples (of the same size). This is taken as evidence that it is unlikely (although still possible) that the observed results arose from chance alone. If the *P*-value is high, it indicates that differences as large as those observed would occur by chance in a high proportion of possible samples, even if there were no "differences" in the underlying population.

In hypothesis testing, the null hypothesis is either accepted or rejected, depending on whether the *P*-value is above or below a predetermined cut-off point, known as the significance level of the test. If the *P*-value is less than the cut-off point, the null hypothesis is rejected. If the *P*-value is greater than or equal to the cut-off point, the null hypothesis is accepted. It is usual to choose either 0.05 (5%) or 0.01 (1%) as significance levels for testing the null hypothesis.

As an example, suppose it is known that in a particular country the weight at birth of male babies is normally distributed with a mean of 3.3 kg and a standard deviation of 0.5. Suppose further that a random sample of 100 male babies born to a particular ethnic subgroup was found to have a mean birth weight of 3.2 kg. We wish to determine whether the mean birth weight in the ethnic subgroup is different from the birth weight in the country as a whole. The null hypothesis would state that the mean birth weight of the ethnic subgroup is 3.3 kg.

In this example, the appropriate test statistic is z:

$$z = \frac{\bar{x} - \mu}{\sigma/\sqrt{n}}$$

where

$\bar{x}$ = sample mean,

μ = known country mean,

σ = known standard deviation,

n = sample size.

For the above example:

$$z = \frac{3.2 - 3.3}{0.5/\sqrt{100}} = -2$$

The statistic z has been constructed so that if the null hypothesis were true (i.e. birth weights in the population sampled were normally distributed with a mean μ and standard deviation σ), then the distribution of z over all possible samples of size n would be close to that of a normal distribution with mean 0 and standard deviation 1. An important characteristic of this distribution is that the area under the normal curve to the right of the line $z = \text{a}$ (see Fig. 4.6) can be interpreted as the probability with which values of z are greater than a. Similarly, the area under the curve to the left of the line $z = -\text{a}$ gives the probability with which values of z are less than $-$ a. Therefore, the P value associated with a particular value $z = \text{a}$, is equal to the area under the normal curve to the right of $z = \text{a}$, *plus* the area under the curve to the left of $z = -\text{a}$.

For the above example, consultation of the appropriate normal distribution tables found in many statistical textbooks (which give P values for areas under the normal curve associated with each value of z) indicates that the area under the curve to the left of $z = -2$ is 0.023. Similarly the area under the curve to the right of $z = 2$ is 0.023. Therefore the P-value associated with this value of z is

Fig. 4.6. Areas under the normal curve

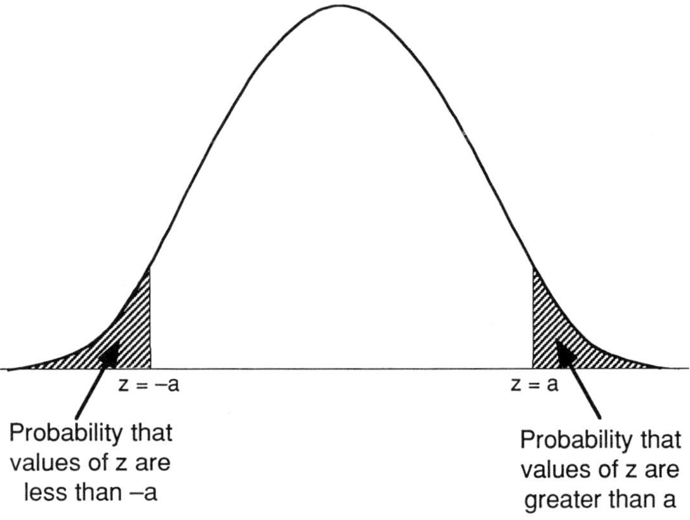

0.046. This can be interpreted as indicating that if the null hypothesis were true (i.e. birth weights in the ethnic subgroup are normally distributed with a mean of 3.3 and standard deviation 0.5), only 4.6% of all possible samples of 100 babies would have mean birth weights differing from 3.3 kg by 100 grams or more.

If we had decided on a significance level of 5% for the statistical test, we would reject the null hypothesis and accept the alternative that the mean of the population is not equal to 3.3. However, had we decided on the 1% level of significance the null hypothesis would have been accepted. The phrase "statistically significant" is used to indicate that a result has led to rejection of the null hypothesis. It is important to keep in mind that the null hypothesis is never proven right or wrong but is only accepted or rejected at a given level of significance. The *P* value is influenced by both the strength of the association and the sample size. A small *P* value may be consistent with a weak association, and a difference between two groups may fail to be statistically significant if the sample size is not large enough (see pages 46–47).

Many statistical tests involve the comparison of two quantities (in the example above, the sample mean was compared with the known country mean). Usually the statistical test allows for the possibility of differences in both directions (either quantity can be larger than the other; the country mean might have been greater than the sample mean or smaller than it). This is known as a two-sided or two-tailed test. As in the example above, the *P* value is calculated on the basis of probabilities from both tails of the sampling distribution. (Thus, in the above example *P* was the sum of the probability of $z > +2$ and $z < -2$.)

However there are some situations in which there is interest in a difference in only one direction. For example, one may wish to test whether a specific treatment is better than a placebo (the case in which the treatment is worse than the placebo being of no interest). In this instance it would be appropriate to use a "one-sided" or "one-tailed" test. The calculation of the test statistic for a one-sided test is identical to that of the two-sided test. The difference between the two types of tests lies in the calculation of the *P* value. A one-sided test is based on probabilities from only one side or one tail of the sampling distribution, whereas a two-sided test sums the probabilities from both tails of the distribution. Therefore the *P* value associated with the one-sided test is equal to half the *P* value associated with the two-sided test.

There are other circumstances in which it could be safely assumed that one quantity would be larger than the other. For example, in a study on the effects of an environmental hazard, data from animal experiments or case series may already have shown the likely consequence of exposure. Prenatal exposure to methylmercury has been shown to cause damage to the central nervous system and developmental disturbance in animals. A study of cerebral palsy in Minamata, Japan, indicated that this syndrome occurred frequently in the children of women who ate fish containing high levels of methylmercury during pregnancy (WHO, 1990). Future epidemiological studies on central nervous system effects of prenatal exposure to methylmercury may therefore be based on the assumption that such exposure is not going to be beneficial to children, and one-tailed statistical tests would be appropriate.

The advantage of a one-tailed test is that the sample size required is smaller than that needed for the same precision in a two-tailed test. However, one-tailed tests should be used only if differences in a single direction are of interest or if one has prior knowledge that differences occur in only one direction. Whichever approach to significance testing is used, the methods and the measuring should be clearly explained in the study plan and report.

Another set of useful statistical tests are known as t-tests, and are especially important for small samples. For instance, one can test the hypothesis that the mean of a population is equal to a predetermined value, μ, when the standard deviation of the underlying population is unknown, but the standard deviation of the sample is known. The appropriate formula is:

$$t = \frac{\bar{x} - \mu}{s/\sqrt{n}}$$

where
s is the standard deviation of the sample
and t has $n - 1$ degrees of freedom.

This is similar to the z-test described above. However, the z-statistic is used when the standard deviation of the population is known, while the t-statistic is used when the standard deviation of the population is unknown and estimated by the standard deviation of the sample.

The t distribution can also be used to test whether the means of two independent samples are significantly different. This test assumes that both samples have been drawn from a single population, or from two populations with equal variance. The test statistic is then:

$$t = \frac{\bar{x}_1 - \bar{x}_2}{s_p\sqrt{(1/n_1) + (1/n_2)}}$$

where $\bar{x}_1$ = mean of first sample,

$\bar{x}_2$ = mean of second sample,

n_1 = sample size of first sample,

n_2 = sample size of second sample,

s_1 = standard deviation of first sample,

s_2 = standard deviation of second sample,

$$s_p^2 = \frac{(n_1 - 1)s_1^2 + (n_2 - 1)s_2^2}{n_1 + n_2 - 2}$$

Other uses of the t distribution include testing whether linear regression and correlation coefficients are significant.

Type I and type II errors

As indicated above, in statistical analysis a hypothesis is never proven to be true or false but is only accepted or rejected on the basis of statistical tests. Two types of error are associated with this decision: to reject the null hypothesis when it is true (this is called a type I error or an alpha error), and to accept the null hypothesis when it is false (this is called a type II error or a beta error). The probability of making a type I error is the level of significance of the statistical test, which should always be stated when results are presented.

For example, randomized clinical trials of drugs can lead to both type I and type II errors. It may be concluded on the basis of the results that a new treatment is effective when in fact it is no better than the standard treatment. This type of error, which leads to a false positive conclusion that the treatment is effective, is a type I error. On the other hand, a new treatment that is actually effective may be concluded to be ineffective. Such a false negative conclusion is a type II error.

The probability of rejecting the null hypothesis when it is false is known as the power of a statistical test. It is equal to one minus the probability of a type II error. The power of a test depends on the sample size—the larger the sample size, the higher the power, all else being equal. The power of a test is also dependent on the significance level chosen. For any given sample size, the higher the level of significance (i.e. the lower the probability of a type I error), the lower is the power (the more likely a type II error will be made). It is common for studies to aim for a power of 0.8 at a significance level of 0.05. This means that the probability of a type II error (0.2) is four times the probability of a type I error (0.05), reflecting the fact that, in most studies, a type I error is considered much more serious than a type II error. The power should be presented when a negative result is reported.

The power of a test is an important consideration in the planning of an epidemiological study, since it indicates how likely the test is to have a statistically significant result under different circumstances.

Differences between statistical, clinical and public health significance

Statistical methods give an estimate of the probability that observed differences between groups are due to chance. Clinical and public health significance, on the other hand, concerns the relevance of findings to clinical or public health practice. Because statistical significance is in part dependent on sample size, it is possible that small and clinically unimportant differences may reach statistical significance. On the other hand, a result that is important from the public health perspective may be overlooked because the study sample is not large enough to reach statistical significance, which means that the study is too small for safe conclusions to be drawn. When judging and interpreting data, epidemiologists must always bear in mind their significance from both the clinical and public health standpoints.

Relationship between two variables

Epidemiological studies are often concerned with evaluating the relationship between two variables. After looking at the distribution of each variable separately, it is useful to make a cross-tabulation of the data, in which the frequencies of both variables are presented in a tabular form. Table 3.4 (page 38) is an example of the cross-tabulation of two nominal variables (presence of enteritis necroticans and ingestion of meat). Interval variables can also be cross-tabulated using interval subgroups.

There are many ways of assessing the association between two variables. Three of the most commonly used methods are described below.

Chi-squared test

When two variables are categorical, the chi-squared (χ^2) test is commonly used to examine the null hypothesis that the distributions of the variables are independent of each other (i.e. that the frequency of falling into a particular category of variable A is the same for all categories of variable B). Table 4.2 shows the distribution of two variables, A and B, and the equation needed to calculate the appropriate χ^2 statistic to test for an association between them.

Table 4.2. Calculation of χ^2 statistic

		Variable A		
		present	**absent**	**Total**
Variable B	**present**	a	b	$a+b$
	absent	c	d	$c+d$
	Total	$a+c$	$b+d$	n

$$\chi^2 = \frac{(|ad - bc| - n/2)^2 n}{(a+b)(a+c)(c+d)(b+d)}$$

For the data in Table 3.4 the null hypothesis would be that the two variables, recent meat ingestion and enteritis necroticans, were independent. For a level of significance of 0.05, the cut-off for the χ^2 value for a 2×2 table is 3.84 (χ^2 tables can be found in elementary statistics books). If the calculated χ^2 value is greater than 3.84, the null hypothesis should be rejected at the 5% level of significance.

Substituting the values from Table 3.4, we find that $\chi^2 = 32.57$. Therefore we reject the null hypothesis and accept the alternative that there is an association between recent meat ingestion and enteritis necroticans.

Correlation

Correlation can be thought of as the degree to which two variables change together. It is measured by the correlation coefficient. Several correlation coefficients are frequently used in epidemiological studies. They all have a range of values between $+1$ and -1, the value zero indicating the absence of correlation, and the values $+1$ and -1 indicating perfect positive and negative correlation respectively. The Pearson product moment correlation coefficient (r) measures the degree of linear relationship between two variables. If there is a perfect linear correlation between two variables, this means that all the observed values lie on a straight line, and $r = 1.0$ or -1.0.

The formula for Pearson's product moment correlation coefficient r for variables x and y is:

$$r = \frac{\Sigma(x_i - \bar{x})(y_i - \bar{y})}{\sqrt{\Sigma(x_i - \bar{x})^2 \, \Sigma(y_i - \bar{y})^2}}$$

It is important to stress that the Pearson product moment correlation coefficient measures the degree of linear relationship only, and that two variables may be highly related in a nonlinear way and have a very low correlation coefficient.

Two other correlation coefficients often used in epidemiology are the Spearman rank-order correlation coefficient (r_s) and the Kendall rank-order correlation coefficient (τ). Both of these coefficients are applicable to ranked data. For an in-depth treatment of these coefficients readers may wish to consult Siegel & Casterllan, 1988.

Regression

Regression analysis can be thought of as finding the best mathematical model for predicting one variable from another. One variable is considered to be a dependent variable, its value varying according to one or more independent variables. The most common form of regression is linear regression, in which the mathematical model is a straight line; the regression equation is the equation of the straight line that best fits the data.

The regression line in Fig. 4.7 is based on data concerning the prevalence of underweight children and the intake of energy per capita from 11 Asian

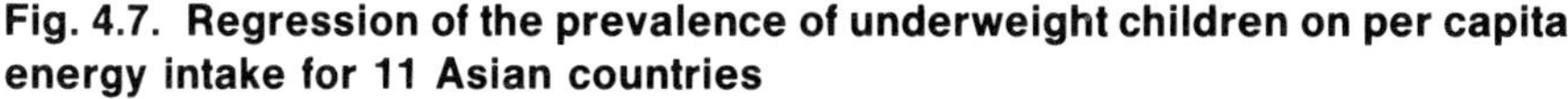

Fig. 4.7. Regression of the prevalence of underweight children on per capita energy intake for 11 Asian countries

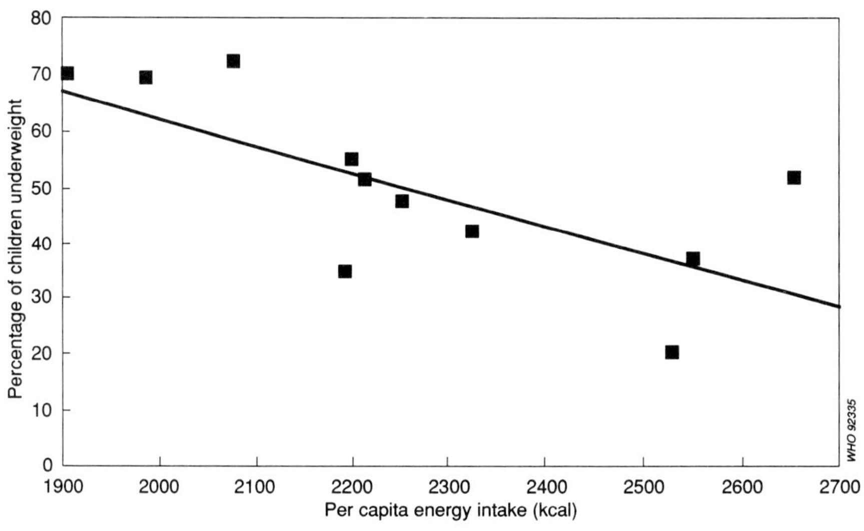

countries. The data indicate that there is a negative linear relationship between these two variables, but as can be seen from the scatter plot, the relationship is far from perfect.

The regression line for this example is: $y = 162.5 - 0.05x$

where y = prevalence of underweight children (%)

x = energy intake per day (kcal).

Although the example given involves only one independent variable, regressions often involve several such variables; this is called multiple regression.

Other commonly used regression models take into consideration the nonlinear relationship between variables: polynomial regression, logistic regression and proportional hazards models are in this category.

Study questions

4.1 Make an estimate of the mean and median of the data in Table 4.1. Why do the mean and median have different values?

4.2 In a study to investigate the therapeutic effects of high and low doses of antidepressant medication, patients were randomly assigned to a low-dosage or high-dosage regimen. They were assessed initially and after 14 and 28 days using standardized rating scales. In comparing the two dosage groups, should one-tailed or two-tailed tests be used? Give reasons.

4.3 Give an example of a situation in which it would be more useful to examine the median of a distribution rather than the mean.

Chapter 5

Causation in epidemiology

A major goal of epidemiology is to assist in the prevention and control of disease and in the promotion of health by discovering the causes of disease and the ways in which they can be modified. Indeed, as was illustrated in Chapter 1, the discipline has had remarkable successes in this respect. The present chapter describes the epidemiological approach to causation.

The concept of cause

An understanding of the causes of disease is important in the health field not only for prevention but also in diagnosis and the application of correct treatments. The concept of cause is the source of much controversy in epidemiology, as it is in other sciences. The philosophy of science continues to make contributions to the understanding of the process by which causal inferences, i.e. judgements linking postulated causes and their outcomes, are made. The concept of cause has different meanings in different contexts and no definition is equally appropriate in all sciences.

A cause of a disease is an event, condition, characteristic or a combination of these factors which plays an important role in producing the disease. Logically, a cause must precede a disease. A cause is termed sufficient when it inevitably produces or initiates a disease and is termed necessary if a disease cannot develop in its absence.

A sufficient cause is not usually a single factor, but often comprises several components. In general, it is not necessary to identify all the components of a sufficient cause before effective prevention can take place, since the removal of one component may interfere with the action of the others and thus prevent the disease. For example, cigarette smoking is one component of the sufficient cause of lung cancer. Smoking is not sufficient in itself to produce the disease: some people smoke for 50 years without developing lung cancer; other factors, mostly unknown, are required. However, the cessation of smoking reduces the number of cases of lung cancer in a population even if the other component causes are not altered.

Each sufficient cause has a necessary cause as a component. For example, in a study of an outbreak of foodborne infection it may be found that chicken salad and creamy dessert were both sufficient causes of salmonella diarrhoea. The occurrence of salmonellae is a necessary cause of this disease. Similarly, there are different components in the causation of tuberculosis, but the tubercle bacillus is a necessary cause (Fig. 5.1). A causal factor on its own is often neither necessary nor sufficient, e.g., smoking as a factor in causing stroke.

Fig. 5.1. Causes of tuberculosis

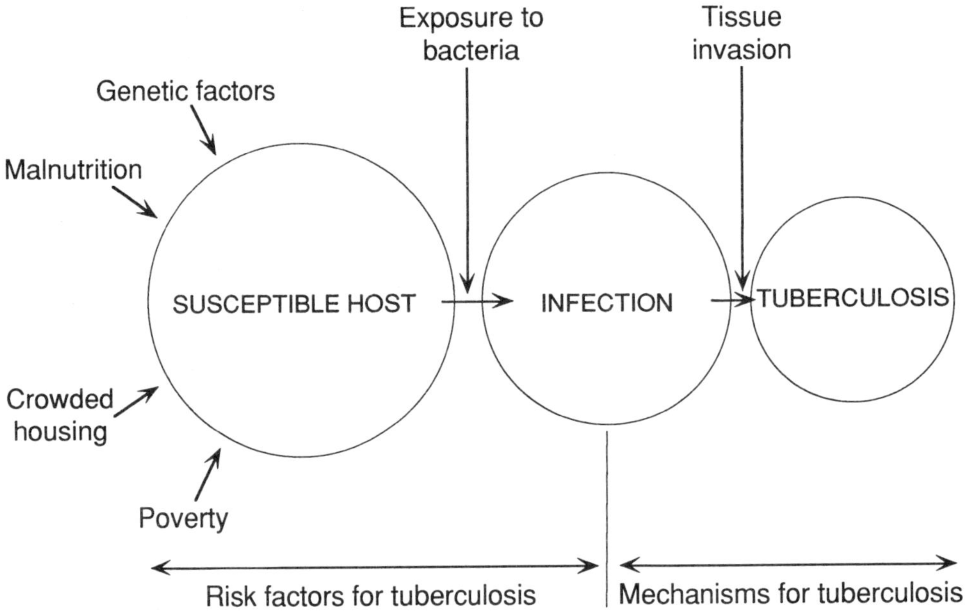

WHO 92336

The usual approach in epidemiology is to begin with a disease and search for its causes, although it is also possible to start with a potential cause (e.g. air pollution) and search for its effects. Epidemiology encompasses a whole set of relationships. For example, social class is associated with a range of health problems. Low social class, as measured by income, education, housing and occupation, appears to lead to a general susceptibility to poor health, rather than to a specific effect. A gamut of specific causes of disease could explain why poor people have poor health, among them excessive exposure to infectious agents due to overcrowding, insufficient food, and dangerous working conditions.

Epidemiologists have been criticized, particularly by laboratory scientists, for not using the concept of cause in the sense of being the sole requirement for the production of disease. Such a restrictive view of causation, however, does not take into account the common multifactorial causation of disease and the need to focus prevention strategies on those factors that can be influenced. Laboratory scientists might, for example, suggest that the basic cause of coronary heart disease relates to cellular mechanisms involved in the proliferation of tissue in the arterial wall. Research directed at determining pathogenic relationships is obviously important, but concepts of causation should be more widely applied than this.

It is often possible to make major progress in prevention by dealing only with the more remote environmental causes. Environmental changes were effective in preventing cholera before the responsible organism, let alone its mechanism of action, had been identified (Fig. 5.2). However, it is of interest that, already in

Fig. 5.2. Causes of cholera

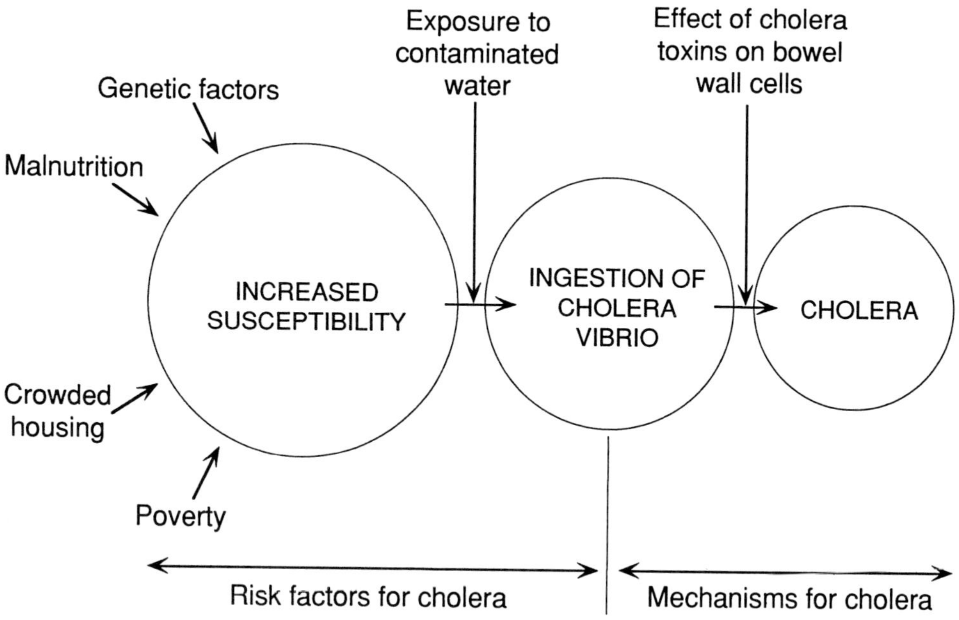

Genetic factors
Malnutrition
Crowded housing
Poverty
INCREASED SUSCEPTIBILITY
Exposure to contaminated water
INGESTION OF CHOLERA VIBRIO
Effect of cholera toxins on bowel wall cells
CHOLERA
Risk factors for cholera
Mechanisms for cholera

WHO 92337

1854, Snow thought that a living organism was responsible for the disease (see page 1).

Single and multiple causes

Pasteur's work on microorganisms led to the formulation, first by Henle and then by Koch, of the following rules for determining whether a specific living organism causes a particular disease:

- the organism must be present in every case of the disease;
- the organism must be able to be isolated and grown in pure culture;
- the organism must, when inoculated into a susceptible animal, cause the specific disease;
- the organism must then be recovered from the animal and identified.

Anthrax was the first disease demonstrated to meet these rules, which have proved useful with some other infectious diseases.

However, for most diseases, both infectious and noninfectious, Koch's rules for determining causation are inadequate. Many causes are usually operating, and a single factor, e.g. cigarette smoking, may be a cause of many diseases. In addition, the causative organism may disappear when a disease has developed, making it impossible to demonstrate the organism in the sick person. Rules such as Koch's are of value only when the specific cause is an overpowering infectious agent, an uncommon situation; susceptibility due to other factors, and a sufficient amount of the agent (the "infective dose"), are usually required before clinical disease develops.

Factors in causation

Four types of factor play a part in the causation of disease. All may be necessary but they are rarely sufficient to cause a particular disease or state.

- *Predisposing factors*, such as age, sex and previous illness, may create a state of susceptibility to a disease agent.
- *Enabling factors* such as low income, poor nutrition, bad housing, and inadequate medical care may favour the development of disease. Conversely, circumstances that assist in recovery from illness or in the maintenance of good health could`also be called enabling factors.
- *Precipitating factors* such as exposure to a specific disease agent or noxious agent may be associated with the onset of a disease or state.
- *Reinforcing factors* such as repeated exposure and unduly hard work may aggravate an established disease or state.

The term "risk factor" is commonly used to describe factors that are positively associated with the risk of development of a disease but that are not sufficient to cause the disease. The concept has been found useful in a number of practical prevention programmes (see, for example, Chigan, 1988). Some risk factors (e.g. tobacco smoking) are associated with several diseases, and some diseases (e.g. coronary heart disease) are associated with several risk factors. Epidemiological studies can measure the relative contribution of each factor to disease occurrence, and the corresponding potential reduction in disease from the elimination of each risk factor.

Interaction

The effect of two or more causes acting together is often greater than would be expected on the basis of summing the individual effects. This phenomenon, called interaction, is illustrated by the particularly high risk of lung cancer in people who both smoke and are exposed to asbestos dust (Table 1.3, page 9); the risk of lung cancer in this group is much higher than would be indicated by a simple addition of the risks from smoking and exposure to asbestos dust.

Establishing the cause of a disease

Causal inference is the term used for the process of determining whether observed associations are likely to be causal; the use of guidelines and the making of judgements are involved. Before an association is assessed for the possibility that it is causal, other explanations, such as chance, bias and confounding, have to be excluded. How these factors are assessed has been described in Chapters 3 and 4. The steps in assessing the nature of the relationship between a possible cause and an outcome are shown in Fig. 5.3.

Fig. 5.3. Assessing the relationship between a possible cause and an outcome

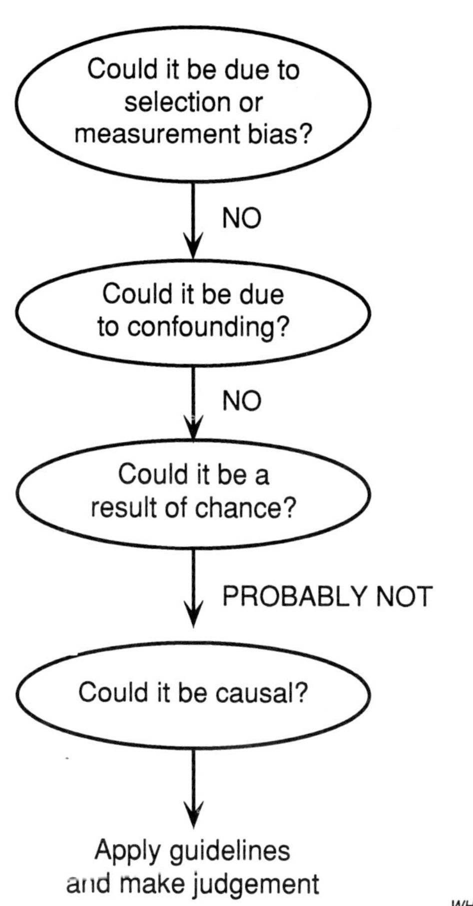

A systematic approach to determining the nature of an association was used by the United States Surgeon General to establish that cigarette smoking caused lung cancer (United States Public Health Service, 1964). This approach was further elaborated by Hill (1965). On the basis of these concepts, a set of "guidelines for causation" has been prepared. In Table 5.1 the concepts are listed in the sequence of testing that the epidemiologist should follow to reach a conclusion about a cause of disease.

Temporal relationship

The temporal relationship is crucial—the cause must precede the effect. This is usually self-evident, although difficulties may arise in case–control and cross-sectional studies when measurements of the possible cause and effect are made at the same time and the effect may in fact alter the exposure (see pages 36 and 37). In cases where the cause is an exposure that can be at different levels, it is

Table 5.1. Guidelines for causation

Temporal relation	Does the cause precede the effect? (essential)
Plausibility	Is the association consistent with other knowledge? (mechanism of action; evidence from experimental animals)
Consistency	Have similar results been shown in other studies?
Strength	What is the strength of the association between the cause and the effect? (relative risk)
Dose–response relationship	Is increased exposure to the possible cause associated with increased effect?
Reversibility	Does the removal of a possible cause lead to reduction of disease risk?
Study design	Is the evidence based on a strong study design?
Judging the evidence	How many lines of evidence lead to the conclusion?

essential that a high enough level be reached before the disease occurs for the correct temporal relationship to exist. Repeated measurement of the exposure at more than one point in time and in different locations may strengthen the evidence.

Fig. 5.4 is an example of a time series of measurements of exposure and effect. It illustrates a sudden increase in the use of seat-belts by car drivers in the United Kingdom after it was made compulsory in January 1983. The incidence of injury decreased simultaneously. As the figures are for total injuries, including both drivers and passengers, they may underestimate the reduction of injury incidence among drivers. The time trends are very suggestive of a protective effect of seat-belts. A cohort study established before 1983 could have measured the effect of seat-belt use more accurately.

Plausibility

An association is plausible, and thus more likely to be causal, if consistent with other knowledge. For instance, laboratory experiments may have shown how exposure to the particular factor could lead to changes associated with the effect measured. However, biological plausibility is a relative concept, and seemingly implausible associations may eventually be shown to be causal. For example, the predominant view on the cause of cholera in the 1830s involved "miasma" rather than contagion. Contagion was not supported by evidence until Snow's work was published; much later, Pasteur and his colleagues identified the causative agent. Lack of plausibility may simply reflect lack of medical knowledge. The scepticism that still exists about the therapeutic effects of acupuncture and homoeopathy may be at least partly attributable to the absence of information about a plausible biological mechanism.

The study of the health consequences of low-level lead exposure is an example of the opposite situation. Animal experiments indicate an effect of lead on the

Fig. 5.4. Frequency of seat-belt use and injury occurrence in the United Kingdom

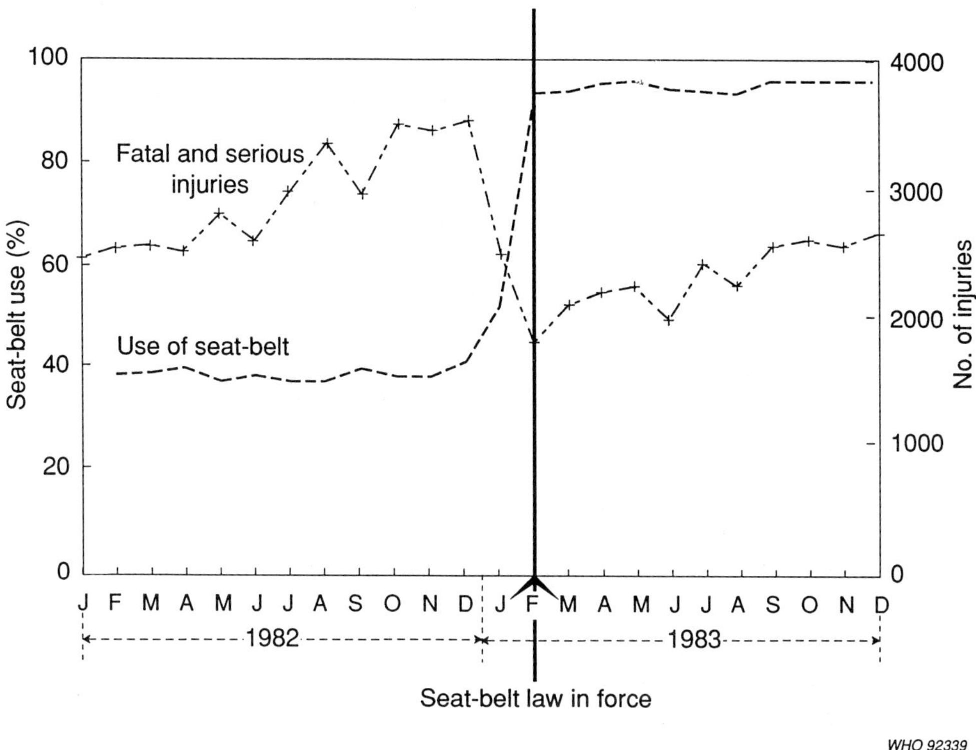

Source: United Kingdom Statistical Service, 1984. Reproduced in *The Quarterly/Journal*, **6**(3): 10 (1984).

central nervous system. Similar effects in an epidemiological study of children are therefore plausible but, because of potential confounding factors and measurement difficulties, epidemiological studies have shown conflicting results. However, assessment of all the available epidemiological data leads to the conclusion that effects do occur in children at a low level of exposure to lead (Mushak et al., 1989).

Consistency

Consistency is demonstrated by several studies giving the same result. This is particularly important when a variety of designs are used in different settings, since the likelihood that all studies are making the same mistake is thereby minimized. However, a lack of consistency does not exclude a causal association, because different exposure levels and other conditions may reduce the impact of the causal factor in certain studies. Furthermore, when the results of several studies are being interpreted the best-designed ones should be given the greatest weight.

Techniques are available for pooling the results of a number of studies that have examined the same issue, particularly randomized controlled trials. Called meta-analysis, this technique combines the results of a number of well-designed trials, each of which may deal with a relatively small sample, in order to obtain a better overall estimate of effect (Sacks et al., 1987).

Fig. 5.5 illustrates the results of 11 trials on the use of β-blockers for the prevention of death after myocardial infarction. One important reason for the apparent inconsistency of the results is that several of the early studies were on small samples. The estimated relative risk in each study is marked by a cross; the horizontal lines indicate the 95% confidence intervals. For the aggregated data from all the trials, covering a very large number of events, the 95% confidence interval is very narrow. Overall, treatment with β-blockers after myocardial infarction is seen to reduce the death rate on average by about 35%; the 95% confidence interval shows that the reduction in death rate is at least 20% and could be as much as 50%.

Fig. 5.5. Meta-analysis of selected randomized trials of beta-blockers in the prevention of deaths following a myocardial infarction

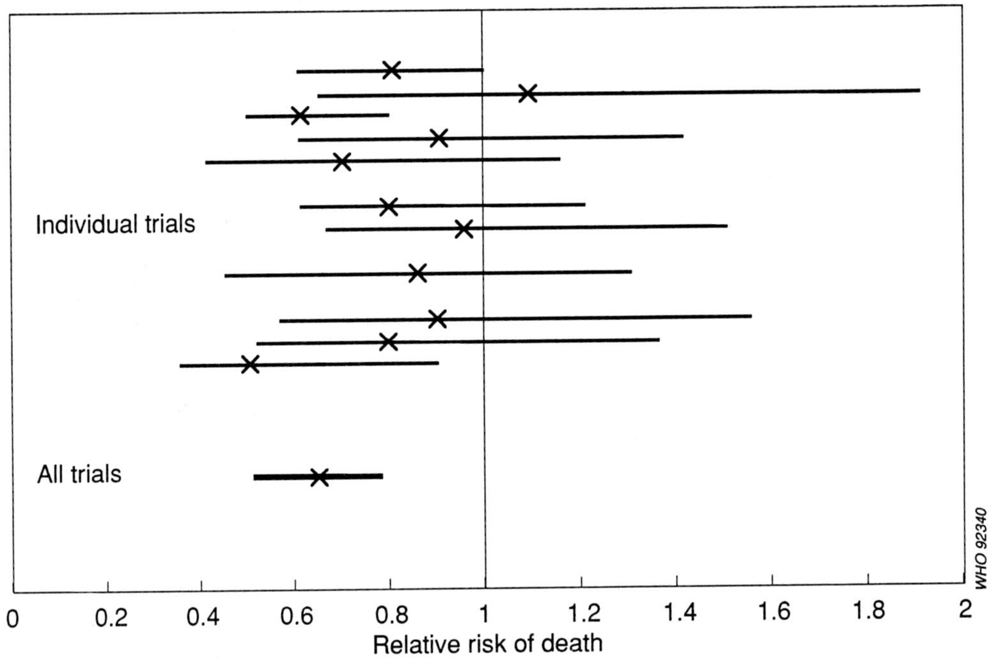

Source: Yusuf et al., 1985. Reproduced by kind permission of the publisher.

Strength

A strong association between possible cause and effect, as measured by the size of the risk ratio (relative risk, see pages 29–30), is more likely to be causal than is a weak association, which could be influenced by confounding or bias. Relative risks greater than 2 can be considered strong. For example, cigarette smokers have an approximately twofold increase in the risk of acute myocardial infarction compared with nonsmokers. The risk of lung cancer in smokers, compared with nonsmokers, has been shown in various studies to be increased between fourfold and twentyfold. However, such very strong associations are rare in epidemiology.

The fact that an association is weak does not preclude it from being causal; the strength of an association depends on the relative prevalence of other possible causes. For example, weak associations have been found between diet and risk of coronary heart disease in observational studies; and although experimental studies on selected populations have been conducted, no fully satisfactory trials have been completed. Despite this, diet is generally thought to be a major causative factor in the high rate of coronary heart disease in many industrialized countries.

The probable reason for the difficulty in identifying diet as a risk factor for coronary heart disease is that diets in populations are rather homogeneous and variation over time for one individual is greater than that between people. If everyone has more or less the same diet it is not possible to identify diet as a risk factor. Consequently, ecological evidence gains importance. This situation has been characterized as one of sick individuals and sick populations (Rose, 1985), meaning that in many industrialized countries whole populations are at risk from an adverse factor.

Dose–response relationship

A dose–response relationship occurs when changes in the level of a possible cause are associated with changes in the prevalence or incidence of the effect (see pages 16–19). Table 5.2 illustrates the dose–response relationship between noise and hearing loss: the prevalence of hearing loss increases with noise level and exposure time.

The demonstration of a clear dose–response relationship in unbiased studies provides strong evidence for a causal relationship between exposure or dose (see page 120) and disease.

Table 5.2. Percentage of people with hearing loss

Average noise level during an 8-hour working day (decibels)	Exposure time (years)		
	5	10	40
< 80	0	0	0
85	1	3	10
90	4	10	21
95	7	17	29
100	12	29	41
105	18	42	54
110	26	55	62
115	36	71	64

Source: WHO, 1980a.

Reversibility

When the removal of a possible cause results in a reduced disease risk, the likelihood of the association being causal is strengthened. For example, the cessation of cigarette smoking is associated with a reduction in the risk of lung cancer relative to that in people who continue to smoke. This finding strengthens the likelihood that cigarette smoking causes lung cancer. If the cause leads to rapid irreversible changes that subsequently produce disease whether or not there is continued exposure (as with HIV infection), then reversibility cannot be a condition for causality.

Study design

The ability of a study design to prove causation is a most important consideration (Table 5.3). The best evidence comes from well-designed, competently conducted randomized controlled trials (page 42). However, evidence is rarely available from this type of study, and usually only relates to the effects of treatment and prevention campaigns. Other experimental studies, such as field and community trials, are seldom used to study causation. Evidence comes most often from observational studies (page 32); almost all the evidence on the health consequences of smoking comes from observational studies.

Table 5.3. Relative ability of different types of study to "prove" causation

Type of study	Ability to "prove" causation
Randomized controlled trials	Strong
Cohort studies	Moderate
Case–control studies	Moderate
Cross-sectional studies	Weak
Ecological studies	Weak

Cohort studies are the next best design because, when well conducted, bias is minimized. Again, they are not always available. Although case–control studies are subject to several forms of bias, the results from large well-designed investigations of this kind provide good evidence for the causal nature of an association; judgements often have to be made in the absence of data from other types of study. Cross-sectional studies are less able to prove causation as they provide no direct evidence on the time sequence of events.

Ecological studies provide the least satisfactory type of evidence on causality because of the danger of incorrect extrapolation to individuals from data on regions or countries (see page 33). However, for certain exposures that cannot normally be measured individually (such as air pollution, pesticide residues in food, fluoride in drinking-water), evidence from ecological studies is very important. Yet only very rarely has it been considered adequate for establishing causation. In 1968 the sale of bronchodilators without prescription in England and Wales was stopped because the increase in asthma deaths in the period 1959–66 had been shown to coincide with a rise in bronchodilator sales. Despite the fact that only very limited evidence was available linking the use of bronchodilators with death in asthmatics, the ecological evidence was deemed sufficient; two decades later this relationship continues to be debated and has relevance to a recent increase in asthma deaths among young people in New Zealand (Crane et al., 1989).

Judging the evidence

Regrettably, there are no completely reliable criteria for determining whether an association is causal or not. Causal inference is usually tentative and judgements must be made on the basis of the available evidence: uncertainty always remains. Evidence is often conflicting and due weight must be given to the different types when decisions are being made. In judging the different aspects of causation referred to above, the correct temporal relationship is essential; once that has been established, the greatest weight may be given to plausibility, consistency and the dose–response relationship. The likelihood of a causal association is heightened when many different types of evidence lead to the same conclusion. Evidence from well-designed studies is particularly important, especially if they are conducted in a variety of locations.

Study questions

5.1 What is causal inference?

5.2 Comment on the statement: "Epidemiology is the only scientific discipline essential to causal inference."

5.3 List the criteria commonly used to assess the causal nature of observed associations.

5.4 A statistically significant association has been demonstrated in a case–control study between the use of a drug for asthma and the risk of dying from asthma in young people. On the basis of this result, would you recommend the withdrawal of the drug?

5.5 During an outbreak of severe neurological disease of unknown cause, the families of the patients suggest that the cause is adulterated cooking oil of a particular brand. Considering the criteria for causality in Table 5.1, what would you try to demonstrate first? What type of study would be suitable? At what stage would you intervene if the accumulating evidence showed that the oil might be the cause?

Chapter 6
Epidemiology and prevention

The scope of prevention

The decline in death rates that occurred during the nineteenth century in the United Kingdom was principally due to a decrease in deaths from infectious disease. A similar decline is now being seen in many developing countries, mainly as a result of general improvements in standards of living, especially in nutrition and sanitation. Significant control of certain diseases has been achieved through specific preventive measures (for example, immunization against poliomyelitis), but in general the role of specific medical therapies has been limited.

Fig. 6.1 shows tuberculosis death rates in England and Wales for the period 1840–1968 and indicates the times of introduction of specific preventive and therapeutic measures. Most of the decline in mortality took place before these

Fig. 6.1. Age-standardized death rates from tuberculosis in England and Wales, 1840–1968

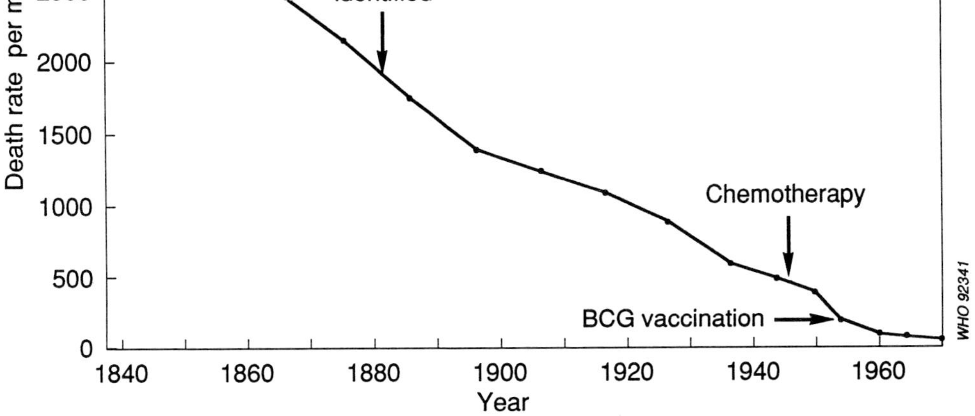

Source: McKeown, 1976. Reproduced by kind permission of the publisher.

interventions and has been attributed to improvements in nutrition and sanitation. The relative contributions of prevention and of medical and surgical interventions to the recent declines in cardiovascular disease mortality in several industrialized countries remain debatable; nevertheless there is strong evidence suggesting that prevention has had the greatest influence.

The changing contributions of chronic and infectious conditions to total mortality in the USA in the period 1900–1973 are shown in Fig. 6.2. In 1900 about 40% of deaths were accounted for by 11 infectious diseases, 19% by three chronic conditions (coronary heart disease, stroke and cancer), 4% by accidents, and the remainder (37%) by all other causes. By the early 1970s, only 6% of deaths were due to the same 11 infectious diseases, 59% were due to the same three chronic conditions, 8% were caused by accidents, and 27% had other causes.

However, changes over time are influenced by the changing age structure of the population, as well as by the waxing and waning of epidemic diseases. The changes in mortality rates over time in developed countries have been particularly dramatic in the youngest age groups, where infectious diseases used to account for most mortality; traffic accidents are now the leading cause of death

Fig. 6.2. Changes in contribution of chronic and infectious conditions to total mortality in the United States, 1900–1973

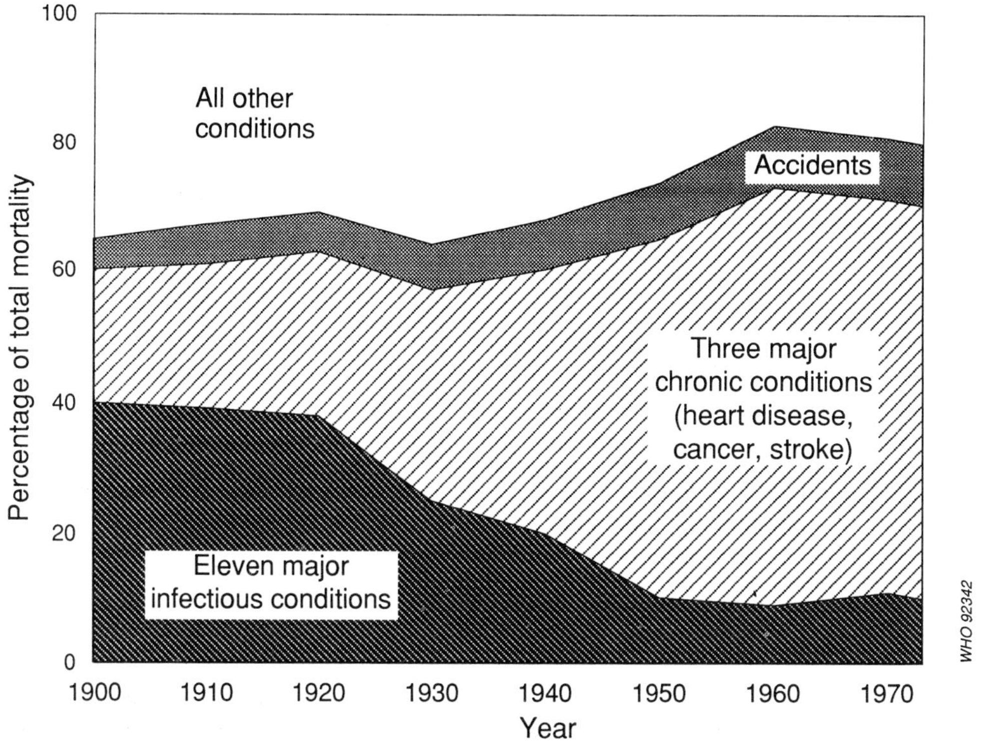

Source: McKinlay et al., 1989. Reproduced by kind permission of the publisher.

in children in many developed countries. The increase in proportionate mortality due to heart disease, cancer and stroke seen in Fig. 6.2 is explained in part by an increase in the number of old people in the population. An analysis of age-specific or age-standardized data is required in order to assess trends properly.

The continuously changing patterns of mortality and morbidity over time in countries indicate that the major causes of disease are preventable. Other evidence of this comes from geographical variation in disease occurrence within and between countries, and from the observation that migrants slowly develop the patterns of disease of host populations. For example, the rates of stomach cancer in people born in Hawaii to Japanese parents are lower than those in Japan (Haenszel et al., 1972). The fact that it takes a generation for the rates to fall suggests the importance of an exposure, such as diet, in early life.

Epidemiology, by identifying modifiable causes of disease, can play a central role in prevention. The many epidemiological studies of coronary heart disease conducted over the past 40 years have identified the size of the problem, the major causes and the appropriate strategies for its prevention and control, thereby contributing to decline in mortality in several countries. In a similar way, epidemiology has helped to reduce the incidences of occupational disease, foodborne disease and injuries sustained in road accidents.

In addition to epidemiologists, other specialists are involved in prevention, among them sanitary engineers, pollution control experts, environmental chemists, public health nurses, medical sociologists, psychologists and health economists. The need for prevention is gaining acceptance in all countries as the limitations of modern medicine in curing disease become apparent and the costs of medical care escalate.

Levels of prevention

Four levels of prevention can be identified, corresponding to different phases in the development of disease (Table 6.1):

- primordial;
- primary;
- secondary;
- tertiary.

All are important and complementary, although primordial prevention and primary prevention have the most to contribute to the health and well-being of the whole population.

Primordial prevention

This level of prevention, the most recent to have been recognized, was identified as a result of increasing knowledge about the epidemiology of cardiovascular diseases. It is known that coronary heart disease occurs on a large scale only if the basic underlying cause is present, i.e., a diet high in saturated animal fat.

Table 6.1. Levels of prevention

Level of prevention	Phase of disease	Target
Primordial	Underlying conditions leading to causation	Total population and selected groups
Primary	Specific causal factors	Total population, selected groups and healthy individuals
Secondary	Early stage of disease	Patients
Tertiary	Late stage of disease (treatment, rehabilitation)	Patients

Where this cause is largely absent, as in China and Japan, coronary heart disease remains a rare cause of mortality and morbidity, despite the high frequencies of other important risk factors such as cigarette smoking and high blood pressure (Blackburn, 1979). However, smoking-induced lung cancer is on the increase and strokes induced by high blood pressure are common in China and Japan.

The aim of primordial prevention is to avoid the emergence and establishment of the social, economic and cultural patterns of living that are known to contribute to an elevated risk of disease. Mortality from infectious diseases is declining in many developing countries and life expectancy is increasing. Consequently, noncommunicable conditions, especially unintentional injuries, cancer and coronary heart disease, take on a greater relative importance as public health problems even before the infectious and parasitic diseases have been fully controlled.

In some developing countries, coronary heart disease is becoming important in the urban middle- and upper-income groups, which have already acquired high-risk behaviour. As socioeconomic development occurs, the risk factors can be expected to become more widespread, leading to major increases in cardiovascular disease.

Primordial prevention is also needed in respect of the global effects of air pollution (the greenhouse effect, acid rain, ozone-layer depletion) and of the health effects of urban smog (lung disease, heart disease). For example, the sulfur dioxide concentrations in the atmosphere in several major cities exceed the maximum recommended by the World Health Organization (Fig. 6.3). Public policies aimed at avoiding the underlying reasons for the development of these hazards are needed in most countries to protect health.

Regrettably, the importance of primordial prevention has often been realized too late. In many countries the basic underlying causes of specific disease are already present, even though the resulting epidemics may still be developing. Cigarette smoking is increasing rapidly in many developing countries, while the overall consumption of cigarettes in many developed countries is dropping (Fig. 6.4). The epidemic of lung cancer may take 30 years to develop in countries newly exposed to cigarette sales promotion. It has been estimated that by 2010 there will be over two million deaths per year in China from smoking-related diseases if a major effort is not made now to reduce smoking (Crofton, 1987).

Fig. 6.3. Summary of annual sulfur dioxide levels in selected cities

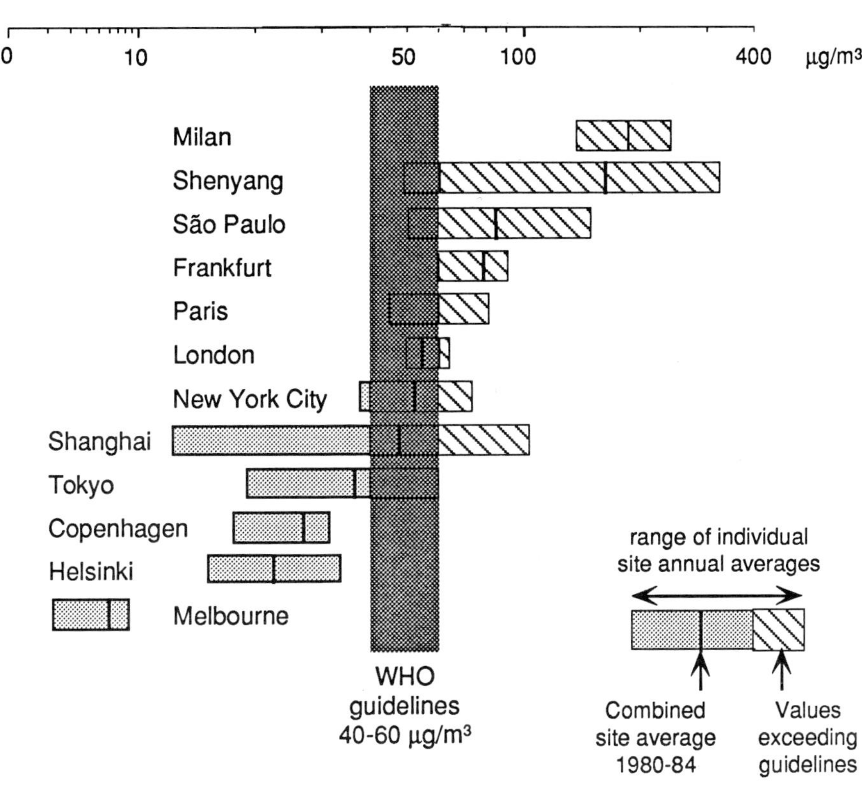

Source: WHO/UNEP, 1988.

Fig. 6.4. Change in total consumption of manufactured cigarettes in six areas, 1970–1985

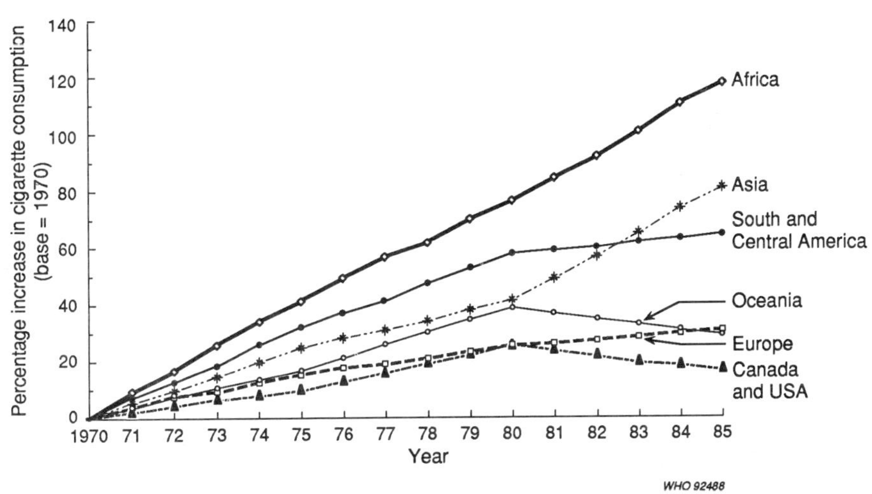

Source: Masironi & Rothwell, 1988.

Effective primordial prevention in this field requires strong government regulatory and fiscal action to stop the promotion of cigarettes and the onset of smoking. Few governments have had the political will to act to prevent epidemics caused by smoking. All countries need to avoid the spread of unhealthy lifestyles and consumption patterns before they become ingrained in society and culture. The earlier the interventions, the more cost-effective they will be (Manton, 1988).

Primordial prevention for coronary heart disease should include: national policies and programmes on nutrition involving the agricultural sector, the food industry, and the food import/export sector; comprehensive policies to discourage smoking; programmes for the prevention of hypertension; and programmes to promote regular physical activity. The example of smoking indicates that a high level of government commitment is required for effective primordial prevention.

Primary prevention

The purpose of primary prevention is to limit the incidence of disease by controlling causes and risk factors. The high incidence of coronary heart disease in most industrialized countries is due to the high levels of risk factors in the population as a whole, not to the problems of a minority. The relationship between serum cholesterol and the risk of coronary heart disease is shown in Fig. 6.5. The distribution of cholesterol is skewed a little to the right. Only a small minority of the population have a serum cholesterol level above 8 mmol/l, i.e. a very high risk of coronary heart disease. Most of the deaths attributable to coronary heart disease occur in the middle range of the cholesterol level, where the majority of the population lies. In this case, primary prevention depends on widespread changes that reduce the average risk in the whole population. The most practical way to do this is to shift the whole distribution to a lower level. This approach is supported by a comparison of the distributions of serum cholesterol in Japan and Finland (Fig. 6.6). There is little overlap: people with high cholesterol levels in Japan would be considered to have low levels in Finland; the death rate from coronary heart disease in Japan is about one-tenth of the rate in Finland. Practical targets for mean serum cholesterol for the purpose of primary prevention have been proposed (Fig. 6.7).

Another example of primary prevention aimed at virtually the whole population is the reduction of urban air pollution through limitation of sulfur dioxide and other emissions from cars, industry and domestic heating. A series of air quality guidelines have been developed (WHO, 1987d) that would lead to primary prevention if enforced. In many cities the guideline values are exceeded (see Fig. 6.3).

A similar approach is applicable in industry, where primary prevention means the reduction of exposure to levels that do not cause ill-health. Ideally, hazards should be totally eliminated; for example benzene, a cancer-causing solvent, has been banned from general industrial use in many countries. If this is not

Fig. 6.5. Relationship between serum cholesterol (histogram) and mortality from coronary heart disease (interrupted line) in men aged 55–64 years

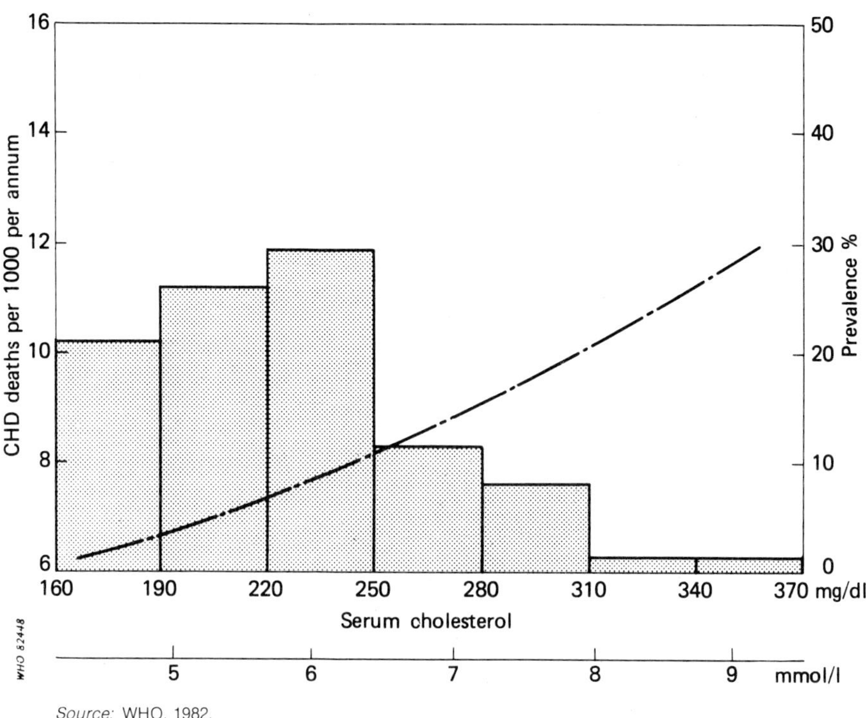

Source: WHO, 1982.

possible, maximum occupational exposure limits can be established and, indeed, have been in most countries.

Further examples of primary prevention are the use of condoms in the prevention of HIV infection, and the development of needle exchange systems for intravenous drug users to prevent the spread of hepatitis B and HIV infection. Education programmes to make people aware of how HIV is transmitted and what they can do to prevent its spread are an essential part of the primary prevention of this disease. Another important way of preventing communicable diseases is to employ systematic immunization, as in the eradication of smallpox.

Primary prevention involves two strategies that are often complementary and reflect two views of etiology. It can focus on the whole population with the aim of reducing average risk (the population strategy) or on people at high risk as a result of particular exposures (the high-risk individual strategy). Epidemiological studies have demonstrated that, although the high-risk individual strategy, which aims to protect susceptible individuals, is most efficient for the people at greatest risk of a specific disease, these people may contribute little to the overall burden of the disease in the population. In this event the population

Fig. 6.6. Distribution of cholesterol levels in Japan and Finland

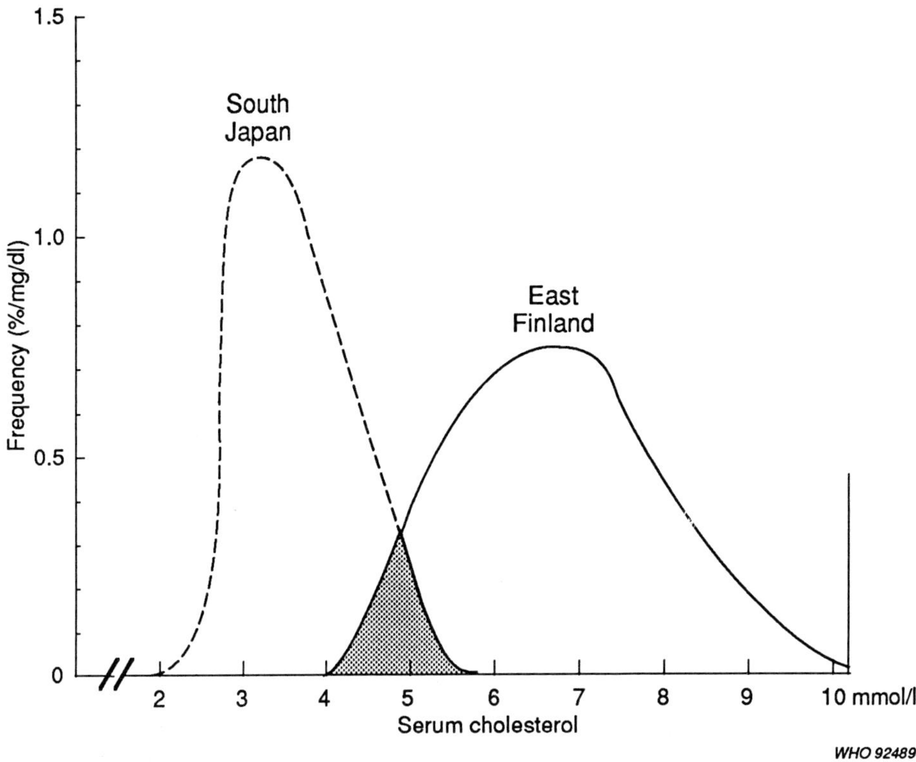

Source: WHO, 1982.

Fig. 6.7. Targets for population mean serum cholesterol levels

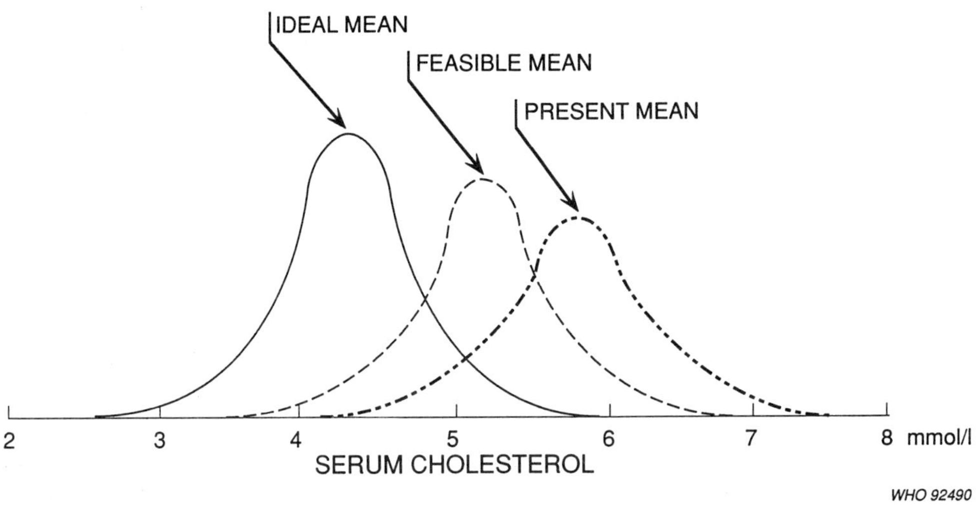

Source: WHO, 1982.

strategy or a combination of both strategies should be applied. The advantages and disadvantages of the two strategies are summarized in Table 6.2.

Table 6.2. Advantages and disadvantages of strategies for primary prevention

Population strategy	High-risk individual strategy
Advantages	
• Radical • Large potential for whole population • Behaviourally appropriate	• Appropriate to individuals • Subject motivation • Physician motivation • Favourable benefit-to-risk ratio
Disadvantages	
• Small benefit to individuals • Poor motivation of subject • Poor motivation of physician • Benefit-to-risk ratio may be low	• Difficulties identifying high-risk individuals • Temporary effect • Limited effect • Behaviourally inappropriate

Adapted from Rose, 1985.

The major advantage of the population strategy is that it does not require identification of the high-risk group. Its main disadvantage is that it offers little benefit to individuals because their absolute risks of disease are quite low. For example, most people will wear a car seat-belt while driving for their entire life without being involved in a crash. The widespread wearing of seat-belts has produced benefits to many societies but little apparent benefit to most individuals. This phenomenon has been called the prevention paradox (Rose, 1985).

With regard to the high-risk strategy, smoking cessation programmes are very appropriate since most smokers wish to abandon the habit and individual smokers and the physicians concerned are usually strongly motivated. The benefits of intervention directed at high-risk individuals are likely to outweigh any adverse effects, such as the short-term effects of nicotine withdrawal. If the high-risk strategy is successful it also brings benefit to nonsmokers by reducing their passive smoking. The disadvantage of the high-risk individual strategy is that it usually requires a screening programme to identify the high-risk group, something that is often difficult and costly.

Secondary prevention

Secondary prevention aims to cure patients and reduce the more serious consequences of disease through early diagnosis and treatment. It comprises the measures available to individuals and populations for early detection and prompt and effective intervention. It is directed at the period between onset of disease and the normal time of diagnosis, and aims to reduce the prevalence of disease.

Secondary prevention can be applied only to diseases in which the natural history includes an early period when it is easily identified and treated, so that progression to a more serious stage can be stopped. The two main requirements for a useful secondary prevention programme are a safe and accurate method of detection of the disease, preferably at a preclinical stage, and effective methods of intervention.

Cervical cancer provides an example of the importance of secondary prevention and also illustrates the difficulties of assessing the value of prevention programmes. Fig. 6.8 shows an association between screening rate and reduction in the death rate from cervical cancer. However, the data have been questioned because the mortality rates for cervical cancer were already decreasing before organized screening programmes started. Other studies support the value of such screening programmes, which are now widely applied in many countries.

Another example is screening for phenylketonuria in newborn children. If children with this condition are identified at birth they can be given a special diet that will allow them to develop normally. If they are not given the diet they become mentally retarded and require special care throughout life. In spite of the low incidence rate of this metabolic disease (2–4 per 100 000 births), secondary prevention screening programmes are highly cost-effective.

Fig. 6.8. Relationship between decrease in death rates from cancer of the cervix between 1960–62 and 1970–72 and population screening rates in several Canadian provinces

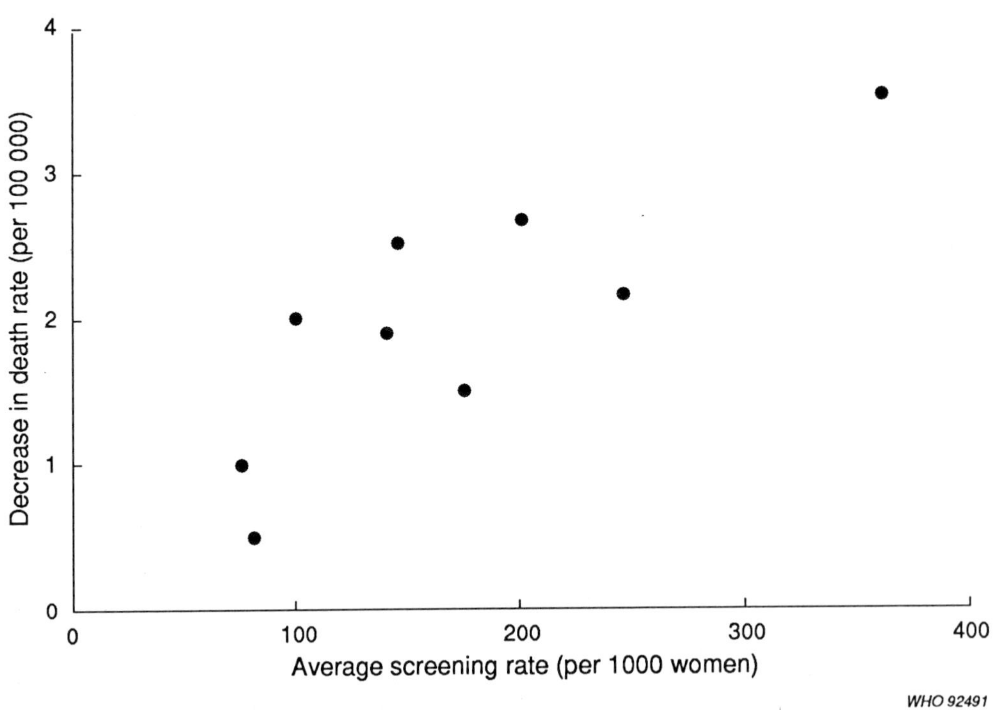

Source: Boyes et al., 1977. Based on data from Miller et al., 1976.

Other examples of secondary prevention measures that are widely used are: blood pressure measurements and treatment of hypertension in middle-aged and elderly people; testing for hearing loss and advice concerning protection against noise in industrial workers; skin testing and chest X-rays for diagnosis of tuberculosis and subsequent treatment.

Tertiary prevention

Tertiary prevention is aimed at reducing the progress or complications of established disease and is an important aspect of therapeutic and rehabilitation medicine. It consists of the measures intended to reduce impairments and disabilities, minimize suffering caused by departures from good health, and promote patients' adjustment to incurable conditions. Tertiary prevention is often difficult to separate from treatment since the treatment of chronic disease has, as one of its central aims, the prevention of recurrences.

The rehabilitation of patients with poliomyelitis, strokes, injuries, blindness and so on is of great importance in enabling them to take part in daily social life. Tertiary prevention can mean a great improvement in individual well-being and family income, in both developed and developing countries.

Screening

Screening is the process by which unrecognized diseases or defects are identified by tests that can be applied rapidly on a large scale. Screening tests sort out apparently healthy people from those who may have a disease. Screening is not usually diagnostic and it requires appropriate investigative follow-up and treatment. Safety is of paramount importance, since the initiative for screening usually comes from the health service rather than from the people being screened.

There are different types of screening, each with specific aims:

- *mass screening* involves the screening of a whole population;
- *multiple* or *multiphasic screening* involves the use of a variety of screening tests on the same occasion;
- *targeted screening* of groups with specific exposures, e.g. workers in lead foundries, is often used in environmental and occupational health;
- *case-finding* or *opportunistic screening* is restricted to patients who consult a health practitioner for some other purpose.

The criteria that should be met before a screening programme is instituted have been described by Wilson & Jüngner (1968). The main ones are listed in Table 6.3. They relate to the characteristics of the disease, its treatment, and the screening test. The disease should be one that would prove serious if not diagnosed early; inborn metabolic defects, such as phenylketonuria, meet this criterion, as do some cancers, e.g. cancer of the cervix.

Table 6.3. Criteria for instituting a screening programme

Disease	Serious High prevalence of preclinical stage Natural history understood Long period between first signs and overt disease
Diagnostic test	Sensitive and specific Simple and cheap Safe and acceptable Reliable
Diagnosis and treatment	Facilities are adequate Effective, acceptable, and safe treatment available

The costs of a screening programme must be balanced against the number of cases detected and the consequences of not screening. Generally, the prevalence of the preclinical stage of the disease should be high in the population screened, but occasionally it may be worthwhile to screen even for diseases of low prevalence which have serious consequences, such as phenylketonuria. The disease must have a reasonably long lead time, i.e. the interval between the time when the disease can be first diagnosed by screening and that when it is usually diagnosed in patients presenting with symptoms. Hypertension has a very long lead time and so has noise-induced hearing loss; pancreatic cancer usually has only a short one. A short lead time implies a rapidly progressing disease and treatment initiated after screening is unlikely to be more effective than that begun after the more usual diagnostic procedures.

Early treatment should be more effective in reducing mortality or morbidity than treatment begun after the development of overt disease, as, for example, in the treatment of cervical cancer *in situ*. A treatment must be not only effective but also acceptable to people who are asymptomatic, and it must be safe. If treatment is ineffective, earlier diagnosis only increases the time period during which the participant is aware of the disease; this effect is known as length bias or length/time bias.

When targeted screening is carried out in groups with particular exposures, the criteria for screening are not necessarily as strict as for general population screening. The health effect that is prevented may be minor (for instance, nausea or headache), but screening may be of high priority if the effect reduces the work capacity and well-being of the patient. This type of screening is common in workplaces. In addition, many health effects arising from exposure to environmental hazards are graded, and the prevention of a minor effect may at the same time prevent more serious effects. Targeted screening is a legal requirement in many countries, for instance, for people working with lead or asbestos, miners, victims of major environmental pollution, and other groups. After the initial screening process more precise tests are used as appropriate.

The screening test itself must be cheap, easy to apply, acceptable to the public, reliable and valid. A test is reliable if it provides consistent results, and valid if it correctly categorizes people into groups with and without disease, as measured by its sensitivity and specificity.

- *Sensitivity* is the proportion of truly ill people in the screened population who are identified as ill by the screening test.
- *Specificity* is the proportion of truly healthy people who are so identified by the screening test.

The methods for calculating these measures and the positive and negative predictive values are given in Table 6.4.

Table 6.4. Validity of a screening test

		Disease status		
		Present	**Absent**	**Total**
Screening test	**Positive**	a	b	$a + b$
	Negative	c	d	$c + d$
	Total	$a + c$	$b + d$	$a + b + c + d$

a = no. of true positives, b = no. of false positives,
c = no. of false negatives, d = no. of true negatives

Sensitivity	= probability of a positive test in people with the disease $= a/(a + c)$
Specificity	= probability of a negative test in people without the disease $= d/(b + d)$
Positive predictive value	= probability of the person having the disease when the test is positive $= a/(a + b)$
Negative predictive value	= probability of the person not having the disease when the test is negative $= d/(c + d)$

Although it would obviously be desirable to have a screening test that was both highly sensitive and highly specific, a balance has to be struck between the two because the cut-off point between normal and abnormal is usually arbitrary. If it is desired to increase sensitivity and to include all true positives, this implies increasing the number of false positives, i.e. decreasing specificity. Reducing the strictness of the criteria for a positive test increases sensitivity but decreases specificity. Increasing the strictness of the criteria increases specificity but decreases sensitivity. Predictive value may also need to be taken into account (see page 111).

Decisions on the appropriate criteria for a screening test depend on the consequences of identifying false negatives and false positives. For a serious condition in newborn children it might be preferable to have high sensitivity and to accept the increased cost of a high number of false positives (reduced specificity). Further follow-up would then be required to identify the true positives and true negatives.

Establishing appropriate criteria requires considerable knowledge of the natural history of the disease in question and of the benefits and costs of treatment. Adequate facilities must exist for formal diagnosis, treatment and follow-up of newly diagnosed cases, which could otherwise overwhelm the health services. Finally, the screening policy and programme must be accepted by all the people involved: administrators, health professionals and the public.

The value of a screening programme is ultimately determined by its effect on morbidity, mortality and disability. Ideally, information should be available on disease rates in people whose disease was identified through screening and in those whose disease was diagnosed on the basis of symptoms. Because differences are likely to exist between people who take part in screening programmes and people who do not, the best evidence for the effectiveness of screening comes from the results of randomized controlled trials. For example, in New York it was found that mammographic screening was effective in reducing mortality from breast cancer in a randomized controlled trial of over 60 000 insured women aged 40–64 which lasted 23 years (Table 6.5). Ten years after entry into the study, the breast cancer mortality was about 29% lower among women who received screening than among the controls; at 18 years, the rate was about 23% lower.

Table 6.5. Breast cancer mortality rates at different times after the start of the follow-up among women receiving screening (mammography) and controls

	No. of women with breast cancer	No. of deaths (from start of follow-up)		
		5 years	10 years	18 years
Screened group	307	39	95	126
Control group	310	63	133	163
% difference		38.1	28.6	22.7

Source: Shapiro, 1989.

Study questions

6.1 Describe the four levels of prevention. Give examples of action at each level which would be appropriate as part of a comprehensive programme to prevent tuberculosis.

6.2 What characteristics of a disease would indicate its suitability for screening?

6.3 What epidemiological study designs can be used to evaluate a screening programme?

Chapter 7

Communicable disease epidemiology

Introduction

A communicable or infectious disease is an illness caused by transmission of a specific infectious agent or its toxic products from an infected person or animal to a susceptible host, either directly or indirectly. Some of the greatest triumphs of epidemiology have stemmed from the prevention and control of communicable diseases, as with Snow's work on cholera and, more recently, the eradication of smallpox.

Communicable diseases continue to present the most important acute health problems in all countries. In developed countries acute upper respiratory tract infections are responsible for a great deal of morbidity and time off work, although only in children and elderly and infirm people are they responsible for significant mortality. In most developing countries, communicable diseases are still the major causes of both morbidity and mortality.

The most striking recent development in this field has been the emergence of new diseases. Lassa fever, a viral disease transmitted from rodents, was first recognized in Nigeria in 1969. Legionnaires' disease, caused by a Gram-negative bacillus, was first described after an outbreak of pneumonia following a meeting of American Legionnaires in Philadelphia in 1976 and was traced to the contamination of air-conditioning equipment. AIDS is the most devastating of the new communicable diseases.

Epidemics and endemic disease

An epidemic is the occurrence in a community or region of a number of cases of a disease that is unusually large or unexpected for the given place and time (Brès, 1986). When an epidemic is described, the time period, geographical region, and particulars of the community group in which the the cases occur must be clearly specified.

The number of cases indicating the presence of an epidemic varies according to the agent, the size and type of population exposed, previous experience or lack of exposure to the disease, and the time and place of occurrence. The identification of occurrence of an epidemic also depends on the usual frequency of the disease in the area among the specified population during the same season of the year. A very small number of cases of a disease not previously recognized in an area, associated in time and place, may be sufficient to constitute an epidemic. For example, the first report on the syndrome that became known as AIDS concerned only four cases of *Pneumocystis carinii* pneumonia in young homosexual men (Gottlieb et al., 1981). Previously this disease had occurred only in

Fig. 7.1. Kaposi sarcoma in New York

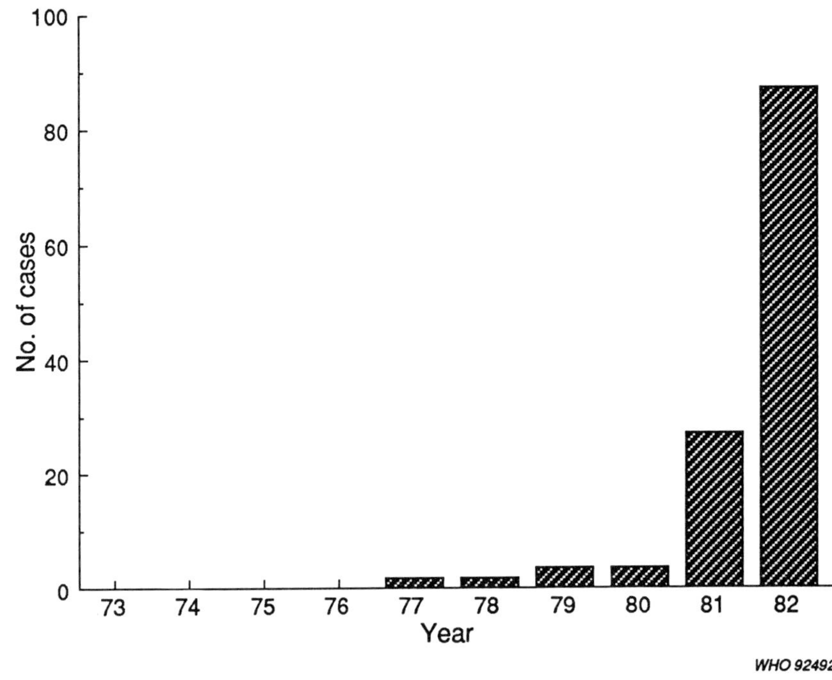

Source: Biggar et al., 1988. Reproduced by kind permission of the publisher.

seriously ill patients with compromised immune systems. The rapid development of the epidemic of Kaposi sarcoma, another manifestation of AIDS, in New York is shown in Fig. 7.1: two cases occurred in 1977 and 1978 and by 1982 there were 88 cases.

Epidemics are usually either point-source or contagious in origin. In a point-source epidemic, susceptible individuals are exposed more or less simultaneously to one source of infection. This results in a very rapid increase in the number of cases, often in a few hours. The cholera epidemic described in Chapter 1 is an example of a point-source epidemic (Fig. 7.2).

In contrast, in a contagious epidemic the disease is passed from person to person and the initial rise in the number of cases is slower. An example is the measles outbreak that occurred among young schoolchildren on a small island in the South China Sea (Fig. 7.3). The children had not been protected by either immunization or previous exposure to measles. The outbreak was small and uncomplicated, and was easily controlled by vaccinating all children. Even so, the economic impact was considerable.

An endemic disease is one that is usually present in a given geographical area or population group at relatively high prevalence and incidence rates, in comparison with other areas or populations. Endemic diseases such as malaria are among the major health problems in developing countries. If conditions change,

Fig. 7.2. Outbreak of cholera, London, August–September 1854

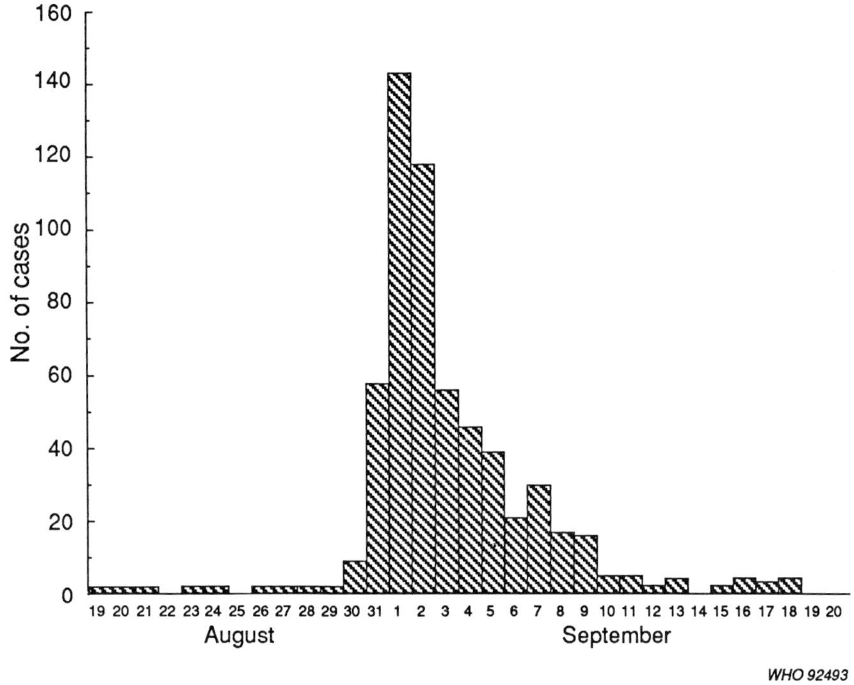

WHO 92493

Source: Snow, 1855.

Fig. 7.3. Measles epidemic in children on a small island

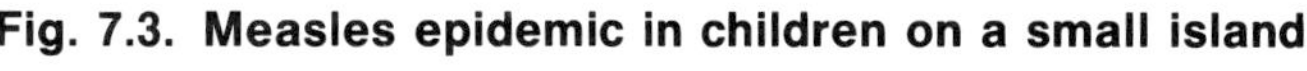

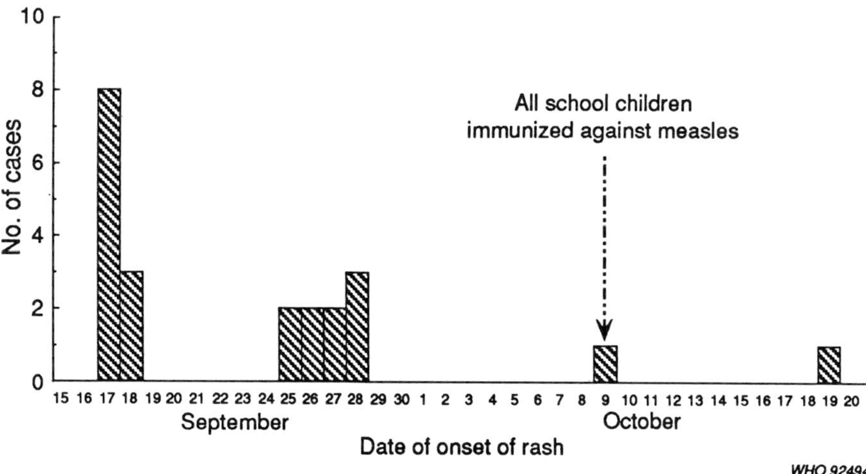

Source: Gao & Malison, 1988. Reproduced by kind permission of the publisher.

either in the host or the environment, an endemic disease may become epidemic. For example, in Europe the reduction in the incidence of smallpox achieved in the early twentieth century was reversed during the First World War (Table 7.1).

Table 7.1. Deaths from smallpox in selected European countries, 1900–1919

	1918 population (millions)	Number of reported deaths 1900–04	1905–09	1910–14	1915–19
Finland	3	295	155	182	1 605
Germany	65	165	231	136	1 323
Italy	34	18 590	2 149	8 773	17 453
Russia	134	218 000	221 000	200 000	535 000[a]

Source: Fenner et al., 1988.
[a] Includes nonfatal cases.

Chain of infection

Communicable diseases occur as a result of the interaction of the agent, the transmission process and the host. The control of such diseases may involve changing one or more of these components, all of which are influenced by the environment. These diseases can have a wide range of effects, varying from inapparent infection to severe illness and death (Fig. 7.4).

Fig. 7.4. The spectrum of illness from communicable disease

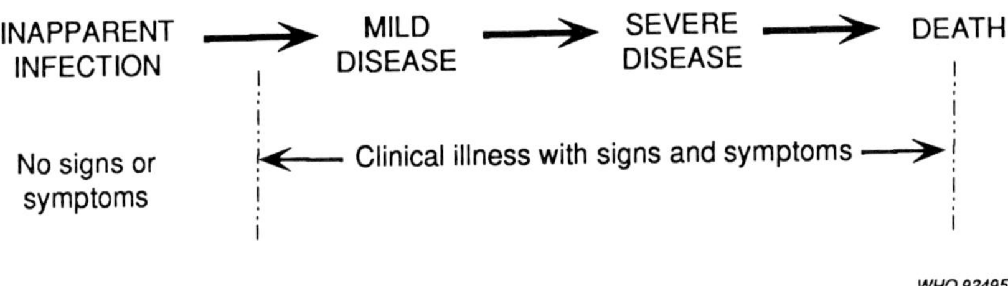

The major thrust of communicable disease epidemiology is to clarify the processes of infection in order to develop, implement and evaluate appropriate control measures. Knowledge of each factor in a chain of infection may be required before effective intervention can take place. However, this is not always necessary; it may be possible to control a disease with only a limited knowledge of its specific chain of infection. For example, improvement of the water supply in London prevented further cholera epidemics 30 years before the responsible agent was identified. Knowledge alone is not sufficient to prevent epidemics, however, and cholera remains an important cause of death and disease in many parts of the world.

The infectious agent

A large number of microorganisms cause disease in humans. Infection is the entry and development or multiplication of an infectious agent in the host. Infection is not equivalent to disease. Some infections do not produce clinical disease. The specific characteristics of each agent are important in determining the nature of the infection, e.g., the types of toxin produced by the agent and its physical structure. The end result of infection is determined by a large number of factors involving all stages in the chain of infection. The *pathogenicity* of the agent, its ability to produce disease, is measured by the ratio of the number of persons developing clinical illness to the number exposed to infection. *Virulence*, a measure of the severity of disease, can vary from very low to very high. Once a virus has been attenuated in a laboratory and is of low virulence, it can be used for immunization, as with the poliomyelitis virus. Infectivity is the ability of the agent to invade and produce infection in the host. The *infective dose* of an agent is the amount required to cause infection in susceptible subjects.

The natural habitat of an infectious agent is called its *reservoir*, and may include humans, animals and environmental sources. The *source* of infection is the person or object from which the host acquires the agent. Knowledge of both the reservoir and the source is necessary if effective control measures are to be developed. An important source of infection may be a carrier, i.e. an infected person who shows no evidence of clinical disease. The duration of the carrier state varies between agents. Carriers can be asymptomatic throughout the course of infection or the carrier state may be limited to a particular phase of the disease. Carriers played a large role in the worldwide spread of the human immunodeficiency virus: in North America, several of the early cases were traced to an airline steward who, of course, travelled widely (Schilts, 1988).

Transmission

This, the second link in the chain of infection, is the spread of an infectious agent through the environment or to another person. Transmission may be direct or indirect (Table 7.2).

Direct transmission is the immediate transfer of the infectious agent from an infected host or reservoir to an appropriate entry point through which human infection can take place. This may be by direct contact such as touching, kissing or sexual intercourse, or by the direct spread of droplets by sneezing or

Table 7.2. Methods of transmission of an infectious agent

Direct transmission	Indirect transmission
Touching	Vehicle-borne (contaminated food, water, towels, farm tools, etc.)
Kissing	Vector-borne (insects, animals)
Sexual intercourse	Airborne, long-distance (dust, droplets)
Other contact (e.g. childbirth, medical procedures, injection of drugs, breast-feeding)	Parenteral (injections with contaminated syringes)
Airborne, short-distance (via droplets, coughing, sneezing)	
Transfusion (blood)	
Transplacental	

coughing. Blood transfusions and transplacental infection from mother to fetus may be other important means of transmission.

Indirect transmission may be vehicle-borne, vector-borne, or airborne. Vehicle-borne transmission occurs through contaminated materials such as food, clothes, bedding and cooking utensils. Vector-borne transmission occurs when the agent is carried by an insect or animal (the vector) to a susceptible host; the agent may or may not multiply in the vector. Long-distance airborne transmission occurs when there is dissemination of very small droplets to a suitable point of entry, usually the respiratory tract. Dust particles also facilitate airborne transmission, for example, of fungal spores.

The distinction between types of transmission is important when methods for control of communicable diseases are being selected. Direct transmission can be interrupted by appropriate handling of the source; indirect transmission requires different approaches, such as the provision of mosquito nets, adequate ventilation, cold storage for foods, the reduction of overcrowding, and a supply of sterile disposable syringes and needles.

Host

The host is the third link in the chain of infection and is defined as the person or animal that provides a suitable place for an infectious agent to grow and multiply under natural conditions. The points of entry to the host vary with the agent and include the skin, mucous membranes, and the respiratory and gastrointestinal tracts.

The reaction of the host to infection is extremely variable, being determined by the interaction of host, agent and transmission factors. Infection may be unapparent or clinical, mild or severe. The incubation period—the time between entry of the infectious agent and the appearance of the first sign or symptom of the disease—varies from a few days (e.g. foodborne infection by salmonella) to years (AIDS).

An important determinant of the outcome of infection is the degree of natural or vaccine-induced resistance or immunity of the host. Immunity develops after an infection, after immunization, or through transmission of maternal antibodies via the placenta. *Immunization* is the protection of susceptible individuals from communicable disease by the administration of a modified living infectious agent (as for yellow fever), a suspension of killed organisms (as for pertussis), or an inactive agent (as for tetanus).

Environment

The environment plays a critical role in the development of communicable diseases. General sanitation, temperature, air pollution and water quality are among the factors that influence all stages in the chain of infection. In addition, socioeconomic factors, such as population density, overcrowding and poverty, are of great importance.

Investigation and control of communicable disease epidemics

Investigation

The purpose of investigating an epidemic is to identify its cause and the best means to control it. This requires detailed and systematic epidemiological work. The investigation involves the following main steps: preliminary investigation; identification of cases; collection and analysis of data; implementation of control measures; dissemination of findings; and follow-up. An investigation often covers several of these steps simultaneously.

The initial stage of investigation should verify the diagnoses of suspected cases and confirm that an epidemic exists. The preliminary investigation also leads to the formulation of hypotheses about the source and spread of the disease and this in turn may lead to immediate control measures. Early reports of a possible epidemic may be based on observations made by a small number of health workers or may reflect figures gathered by the formal communicable disease notification system that operates in most countries. Sometimes reports from several health districts are needed: the number of cases in a single area may be too small to draw attention to an epidemic.

Surveillance is an essential part of disease control. There are a number of ways of undertaking surveillance for communicable disease control, the most important being a routine system of reporting cases within the health system. It requires continuing scrutiny of all aspects of the occurrence and spread of disease, generally using methods distinguished by their practicability, uniformity and, frequently, their rapidity, rather than by complete accuracy. The analysis of data from a surveillance system indicates whether there has been a significant increase in the reported number of cases. In many countries, unfortunately, surveillance systems are inadequate, particularly if they depend on voluntary notification.

Sentinel health information systems, in which a limited number of general practitioners report on a defined list of carefully chosen topics that may be changed from time to time, are increasingly used to provide supplementary information for the surveillance of both communicable and noncommunicable diseases. A sentinel network keeps a watchful eye on a sample of the population by supplying regular, standardized reports on specific diseases and procedures in primary health care. Regular feedback of information occurs and the participants usually have a permanent link with researchers.

The investigation of a suspected epidemic requires that new cases be systematically identified, and this means that what constitutes a case must be clearly defined. Often, detailed information on at least a sample of the cases needs to be collected. The cases reported early in an epidemic are often only a small proportion of the total; a thorough count of all cases is necessary to permit a full description of the extent of the epidemic. As soon as an epidemic is confirmed, the first priority is to control it. In severe contagious epidemics, it is often necessary to follow up contacts of reported cases to ensure the identification of all cases and limit the spread of the disease.

Management and control

The management of an epidemic involves treating the cases, preventing further spread of the disease, and monitoring the effects of control measures. Treatment is straightforward except in large-scale epidemics, especially when they occur as a result of social or environmental disruption, when external resources may be needed. The public health action required in emergencies caused by epidemics of different diseases has been described in detail (Brès, 1986).

Control measures can be directed against the source and spread of infection and towards protecting people exposed to it. Usually all of these approaches are required. In some cases, however, removing the source of infection may be all that is necessary, as when a contaminated food is withdrawn from sale. An essential component of control measures is to inform health professionals and the public of the likely causes, the risk of contracting the disease, and the essential control steps. This is particularly important if exposed people have to be protected through either immunization or chemotherapy, e.g. in containing an outbreak of meningococcal meningitis.

Once control measures have been implemented, surveillance must continue to ensure their acceptability and effectiveness. This may be relatively easy in short-term acute epidemics but difficult when dealing with longer-term epidemics, of meningococcal meningitis for example, which require large-scale immunization programmes. Follow-up epidemiological and laboratory studies may be indicated. Thus in low-dose (and therefore relatively cheap) hepatitis B immunization programmes, it may be necessary to conduct long-term investigations before their value can be established.

Systematic immunization programmes can be very effective. For example, on the basis of success in many developed countries, WHO is now calling for the global eradication of poliomyelitis by the year 2000 (WHO, 1989b). The application of epidemiological methods to the investigation and control of epidemics of communicable diseases still presents a challenge to health professionals. Investigation must be undertaken quickly and often with limited resources. The consequences of a successful investigation are rewarding, but failure to act effectively can be damaging. The history of the AIDS epidemic in the USA illustrates both the value and the limitations of epidemiology in this context. By the end of 1982, one year after the publication of the first scientific paper on the new disease, epidemiologists at the Centers for Disease Control in the USA had a clear picture of the nature of the epidemic and the appropriate control measures, although many details had still to be worked out. Since then, vigorous efforts to control AIDS have been made at both the national and global levels; education programmes are essential because AIDS can be controlled only if individuals take preventive actions. Epidemiology thus made a major contribution to understanding of the AIDS pandemic; however knowledge alone is no guarantee that the appropriate preventive actions will be taken.

Study questions

7.1 The contribution of infectious disease to total mortality in the USA during the period 1900–1973 is shown in Fig. 6.2. What possible explanations are there for the change observed?

7.2 If you were a district health officer, how would you monitor the occurrence of measles and detect an epidemic in your district?

7.3 Describe the chain of infection for foodborne disease caused by salmonella.

Chapter 8
Clinical epidemiology

Introduction

Clinical epidemiology is the application of epidemiological principles and methods to the practice of clinical medicine. Of relatively recent origin, the discipline is still refining methods developed primarily in epidemiology and integrating them with the science of clinical medicine. Clinical epidemiology is one of the basic medical sciences, although in most medical schools this is not yet recognized. It includes the methods used by clinicians to audit the processes and outcomes of their work.

It has been suggested that "clinical epidemiology" is a contradiction in terms: epidemiology deals with populations while clinical medicine deals with individuals. This apparent conflict is resolved when it is appreciated that clinical epidemiology works with a defined population of patients rather than with a community-based population. There is no doubt that epidemiology plays an important role in improving the clinical practice of medical practitioners, nurses, physiotherapists and many other health professionals. The justification for the discipline is that clinical decision-making should be based on sound scientific principles; this requires, among other things, relevant research with a strong epidemiological basis.

The central concerns of clinical epidemiology are: definitions of normality and abnormality; accuracy of diagnostic tests; natural history and prognosis of disease; effectiveness of treatment; and prevention in clinical practice.

Definitions of normality and abnormality

The first priority in any clinical consultation is to determine whether the patient's symptoms, signs or diagnostic test results are normal or abnormal. This is necessary before further action can be taken, whether this be investigation, treatment or observation. It would be easy if there were always a clear distinction between the frequency distributions of observations on normal and abnormal people. Regrettably this is rarely so, except in genetic disorders determined by a single dominant gene. Occasionally the frequency distributions overlap, but more often there is only one distribution and the so-called abnormal people are at the tail end of the normal distribution. In this situation three types of criteria have been used to help clinicians make practical decisions.

Normal as common

The criterion usually used in clinical practice is to consider frequently occurring values as normal and those occurring infrequently as abnormal. An arbitrary cut-off point on the frequency distribution (often two standard deviations above or below the mean) is assumed to be the limit of normality; all values beyond this point are considered abnormal. This is called an operational definition of abnormality. If the distribution is in fact Gaussian (normal in the statistical sense) this cut-off point would identify 2.5% of the population as abnormal. An alternative approach, which does not assume a statistically normal distribution, is to use percentiles: the 95th percentile point is often considered the dividing line between normal and abnormal, thus identifying 5% of the population as abnormal.

A major limitation of this criterion for normality is that for most variables there is no biological basis for using an arbitrary cut-off point as a pointer to abnormality. Thus for serum cholesterol or blood pressure there is an increasing risk of cardiovascular disease with increasing levels. Even within the normal ranges, as determined statistically, there is an increased risk of disease compared with lower levels. The majority of coronary heart disease deaths occur at levels of serum cholesterol that are usual; only a small proportion of cases occur at extremely high values (see Fig. 6.5, page 89).

Abnormality associated with disease

A second criterion is based on the distribution of observations for both healthy and diseased people, and attempts to define a cut-off point that clearly separates the two groups. A comparison of the two frequency distributions often shows considerable overlap, as is illustrated by serum cholesterol distributions for people with and without coronary heart disease; choosing a cut-off point that neatly separates cases from non-cases is clearly impossible (see Fig. 8.1). There are always some healthy people on the abnormal side of the cut-off point, and some true cases on the normal side.

These two types of classification error can be expressed quantitatively in terms of the sensitivity and specificity of a test, as discussed on page 95. Sensitivity is the proportion of truly diseased people who are categorized as abnormal by the test. Specificity is the proportion of truly normal people categorized as normal by the test. A balance always has to be struck between sensitivity and specificity; increasing one reduces the other.

Abnormal as treatable

The difficulties in distinguishing between normal and abnormal using the above criteria have led to the use of criteria determined by evidence from randomized controlled trials, which indicate the level at which treatment does more good than harm. Unfortunately this information is only rarely available in clinical practice.

The treatment of elevated blood pressure provides a good example of both the advantages and limitations of this type of criterion (Collins et al., 1990). Early clinical trials provided firm evidence that treating sustained very high diastolic blood pressure ($\geqslant 120$ mmHg) was beneficial. Subsequent trials have indicated

Fig. 8.1. Percentage distribution of serum cholesterol levels (mmol/l) in men aged 50–62 who did or did not subsequently develop coronary heart disease

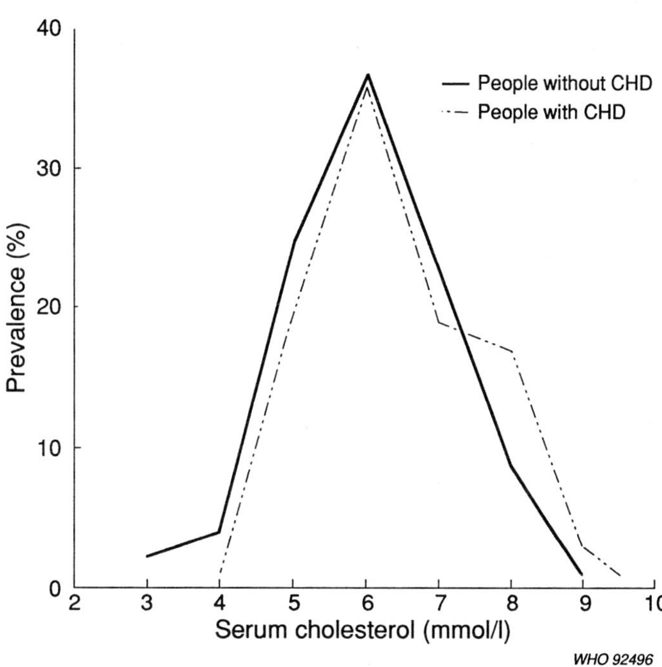

Source: Rose, 1985. Reproduced by kind permission of the publisher.

that the benefits of treatment outweigh the problems at lower levels, perhaps as low as 95 mmHg, which is now the recommended level for treatment in many countries. However, this approach does not take into account the economic and other costs of treatment and is thus still rather simplistic. With the development and application of sophisticated cost–effectiveness analyses it may be possible to bring the cost dimension into clinical decisions. It may soon be feasible to determine blood pressure levels for men and women in specific age groups at which treatment makes economic as well as medical sense. The treatment of a young woman with a diastolic blood pressure of 90 mmHg, who is at low risk of cardiovascular disease, will be much less cost-effective than treating an older man with a diastolic blood pressure of 105 mmHg who has a much greater risk of cardiovascular disease.

What is considered treatable changes with time; this is illustrated by the changing definition of treatable levels of blood pressure (Fig. 8.2). As new evidence accumulates from well-conducted clinical trials, the levels recommended for treatment will continue to change. Each new cut-off point proposed has, however, important logistic and cost implications that need to be considered. The results of the most recent trial of the Medical Research Council in the United Kingdom have suggested that overtreatment might be occurring and there is now a tendency to move treatment levels upwards (Medical Research Council Working Party, 1985).

Fig. 8.2. Treatment of hypertension: changing definition of recommended treatment level over time

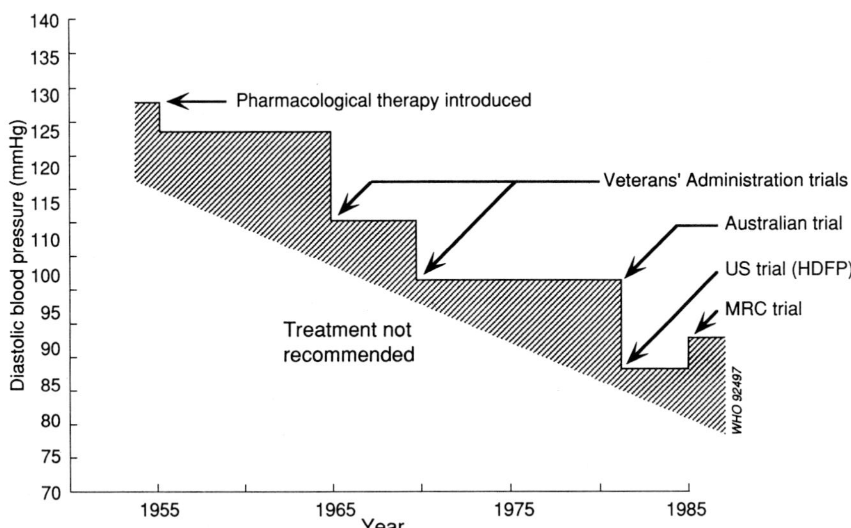

Diagnostic tests

The first objective in a clinical situation is to diagnose any treatable disease present. The purpose of diagnostic testing is to help in confirming possible diagnoses suggested by, for example, the demographic features and symptoms of the patient. In this sense, diagnosis is, or should be, a scientific process, although it is not always clear whether the clinician is attempting to verify or disprove a hypothesis. While diagnostic tests usually involve laboratory investigations (microbiological, biochemical, physiological or anatomical), the principles that help to determine the value of these tests should also be applied to assessing the diagnostic value of symptoms and signs.

Value of a test

A disease may be either present or absent and a test result either positive or negative. There are thus four possible combinations of disease status and test result, as shown in Fig. 8.3 and described in relation to screening tests on page 95.

In two of these combinations the test has given correct answers (true positive and true negative) and in the other two situations it has given wrong answers (false positive and false negative). This categorization can only be made when there is some absolutely accurate method of determining the presence or absence of disease, against which the accuracy of other tests can be determined. Rarely is such a method available, particularly where noncommunicable diseases are concerned. For this reason and because wholly accurate tests are likely to be

Fig. 8.3. Relationship between a diagnostic test result and the occurrence of disease

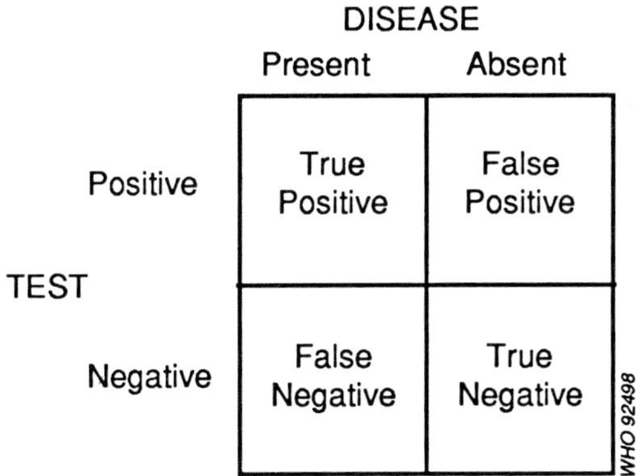

expensive and invasive, simpler and cheaper tests are used in routine clinical practice. However, it is essential that the validity, accuracy and precision of these everyday tests be determined.

Knowledge of other characteristics of tests is also essential in determining their practical usefulness. Of particular importance are a test's positive and negative predictive values, the former being the probability of disease in a patient with an abnormal test result, while the negative predictive value is the probability of a patient not having a disease when the test result is negative.

Predictive value depends on the sensitivity and specificity of the test and, most importantly, on the prevalence of the disease in the population being tested. Even with a high sensitivity and high specificity, if the prevalence is low the positive predictive value of a test may be very low. Given the wide variation in prevalence, this is a more important determinant of the value of a test than sensitivity and specificity.

Natural history and prognosis

The term natural history refers to the stages of a disease, which include:

- pathological onset;
- the presymptomatic stage from onset of pathological changes to the first appearance of symptoms or signs;
- the stage when the disease is clinically obvious and may be subject to remissions and relapses, regress spontaneously, or progress to death.

Detection and treatment at any stage can alter the natural history of a disease, but the effects of treatment can only be determined if the natural history of the disease in the absence of treatment is known.

Prognosis is the prediction of the course of a disease and is expressed as the probability that a particular event will occur in the future. Predictions are based on defined groups of patients and the outcome may be quite different for individual patients. However, knowledge of the likely prognosis is helpful in determining the most useful treatment. Prognostic factors are characteristics associated with outcome in patients with the disease in question. For example, in a patient with acute myocardial infarction, the prognosis is directly related to heart muscle function.

Epidemiological information is necessary to provide sound predictions on prognosis and outcome. Clinical experience alone is inadequate for this purpose since it is often based on a limited set of patients and inadequate follow-up. For example, patients who are seen by a doctor are not necessarily representative of all patients with a particular disease. Patients may be selected according to severity or other features of their disease, or by demographic, social or personal characteristics of the patients themselves. Furthermore, since many doctors do not systematically follow up their patients, they have a limited, and often excessively pessimistic, view of the prognosis of disease. For these reasons epidemiological studies are required to describe accurately the natural history and prognosis of disease.

Ideally, the assessment of prognosis should include measurement of all clinically relevant outcomes, not just death, since patients are usually as interested in the quality of life as they are in its duration. In studies to determine natural history and prognosis, the group of patients should be randomly selected, otherwise selection bias may severely affect the information obtained. For example, the prognosis of patients with chest pain admitted to hospital is likely to be worse than that of patients with chest pain seen by health workers in the community.

Fig. 8.4. Survival following myocardial infarction, Auckland, 1974 and 1981

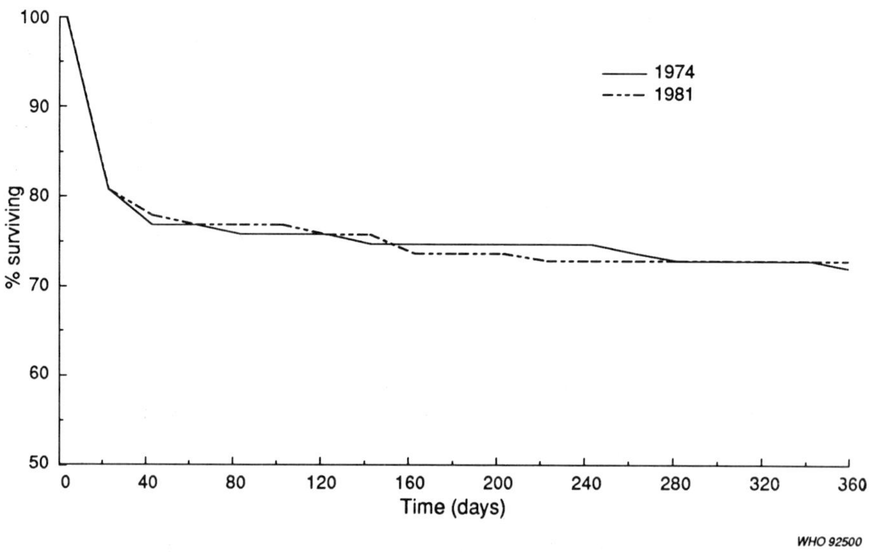

100
90
80
70
60
50
% surviving
—— 1974
---- 1981
0 40 80 120 160 200 240 280 320 360
Time (days)
WHO 92500

Source: Stewart et al., 1984. Reproduced by kind permission of the publisher.

Prognosis in terms of mortality is measured as case-fatality rate or probability of survival. Both the date of onset and the duration of follow-up must be clearly specified. Survival analysis is a simple method of measuring prognosis. The pattern of survival following acute myocardial infarction is shown in Fig. 8.4. Approximately 70% of patients were alive at the end of the first year, most deaths having occurred immediately after infarction. There was no major difference in survival between the groups studied in 1974 and in 1981, despite the efforts directed towards secondary prevention of coronary heart disease.

Life-table analysis is a more sophisticated method that attempts to predict the onset of events over time from previous patterns for all patients at risk. In the follow-up of cohorts of patients to determine prognosis, bias can arise from the method of assembling the cohort and from incomplete follow-up. For example, in the Brazilian cohort of newborn children described on page 40, completeness of follow-up varied according to the income level of the mother.

Effectiveness of treatment

Some treatments are so clearly advantageous that they require no formal assessment; this is true of antibiotics for pneumonia and surgery for serious trauma. However, this situation is relatively rare in clinical medicine. Usually the effects of treatment are much less obvious and most interventions require research to establish their value. Not only must specific interventions be shown to do more good than harm among patients who use them (i.e. they are theoretically effective or *efficacious*), but they should also do more good than harm in patients to whom they are offered (i.e. they should be practically *effective*).

In studies of efficacy it is advantageous to include only patients who are likely to be compliant. *Compliance* is the extent to which patients follow medical advice. Practical effectiveness is determined by studying outcome in a group of people offered treatment, only some of whom will be compliant. From a practical point of view, effectiveness is a more useful measure than efficacy.

The most desirable method for measuring efficacy and effectiveness is that of the randomized controlled clinical trial, as described on pages 42–44. However, there are many situations in which such trials cannot be used and only a small proportion of current medical interventions have been assessed on this basis.

Prevention in clinical practice

Sound epidemiological knowledge encourages the practice of prevention in the context of ordinary clinical practice. Much of this prevention is at the secondary or tertiary level but primary prevention can also be implemented on a routine basis (see Chapter 6). Paediatricians have long been aware of this through their involvement, for example, in child immunization programmes, screening for inborn metabolic defects such as phenylketonuria, and the regular weighing of children and use of standard growth charts. Antenatal care is another good

Fig. 8.5. Self-reporting of stopping smoking at one year follow-up

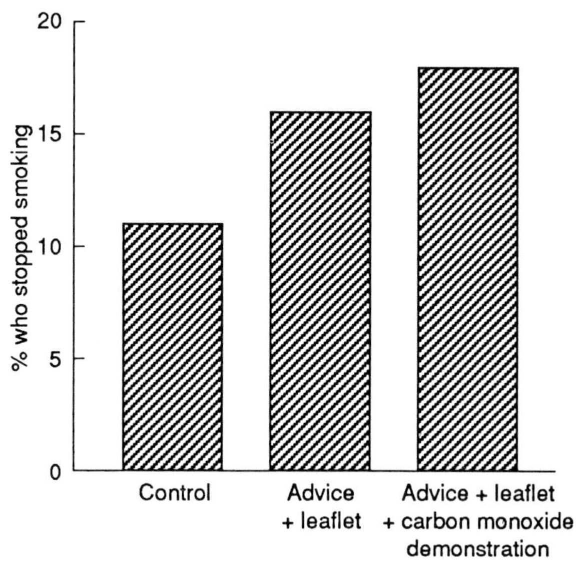

Source: Jamrozik et al., 1984. Reproduced by kind permission of the publisher.

example of the integration of prevention into routine clinical practice, whether by a medical practitioner or some other health professional.

It has been demonstrated that health workers can convince at least some of their patients to stop smoking. A controlled trial of different anti-smoking interventions in general practice showed that advice given routinely against smoking has a useful effect, and that its effectiveness can be improved by using a variety of techniques (see Fig. 8.5). If all health workers were able to achieve even a small level of success in reducing cigarette smoking the impact on the health of the population would be substantial.

Study questions

8.1 Why has the term "clinical epidemiology" been described as a contradiction in terms?

8.2 A commonly used definition of abnormality is based on the frequency of values occurring in a population. What are the limitations of this definition?

8.3 In the table opposite, the results of a new diagnostic test for cancer are compared with the complete diagnostic package in current use. What are the sensitivity and specificity of the new test? Would you recommend its general use?

		Complete diagnosis (true disease status)	
		Disease present	Disease absent
New test	Positive	8	1000
	Negative	2	9000

8.4 What determines the positive predictive value of a screening test?

Chapter 9
Environmental and occupational epidemiology

Environment and health

The human environment consists of very basic elements: the air we breathe, the water we drink, the food we eat, the climate surrounding our bodies, and the space available for our movements. In addition, we exist in a social and spiritual environment, which is of great importance for our mental and physical health.

Most diseases are either caused or influenced by environmental factors. An understanding of the ways in which specific environmental factors can interfere with health is therefore of crucial importance for prevention programmes. Environmental epidemiology provides a scientific basis for studying and interpreting the relationships between environment and health in populations. Occupational epidemiology deals specifically with environmental factors in the workplace. The environmental factors that can cause or contribute to disease are classified in Fig. 9.1.

In a broad sense every disease is caused either by environmental factors or by genetic factors, the latter including natural deterioration of the body with age. The relative contributions of the different factors to the overall morbidity and mortality in a community are difficult to measure, since the major diseases have multifactorial causation. Various estimates for certain disease types and certain factors have been published. For instance, it has been estimated that 80% of all cancers are caused by environmental factors (including tobacco smoking and diet). The interpretation of these types of estimate needs to take into account the age distributions of the diseases under consideration. A cancer occurring in a person aged 85 does not have the same impact on the community and its health status as one affecting someone aged 35.

In epidemiological studies of environmental factors, each factor is often analysed in isolation. It should be remembered, however, that there are many ways in which environmental factors can influence each other's effects. This may explain differences between the results of observational epidemiological studies conducted in different places. The effect of an environmental factor in an individual is also very much dependent on the characteristics of the individual, such as age, sex and physical condition (Fig. 9.2).

The methods used in studies of occupational and general environmental factors are the same as in other branches of epidemiology. However, an important feature of most occupational epidemiology is that it usually deals with an adult population that is young or middle-aged, and often predominantly male. Furthermore, in occupational epidemiology most exposed groups are relatively healthy, at least when they start working. This has given rise to the term

Fig. 9.1. Environmental factors that may affect health

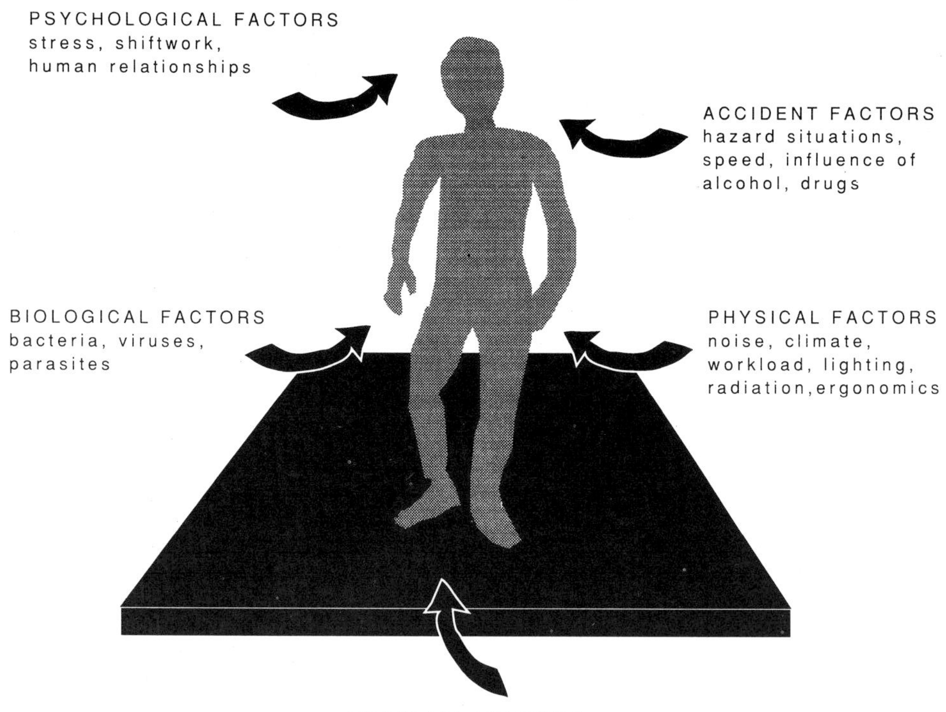

"healthy worker effect", which indicates that the working population has a lower total morbidity and mortality than the population as a whole (see page 48).

In contrast, epidemiological studies of factors in the general environment would normally include children, elderly people and sick people. This is of great importance when the results of occupational epidemiology studies are used to establish safety standards for specific environmental hazards. Exposed people in the general population are likely to be more sensitive than workers in industry. For instance, the effects of lead occur at lower exposure levels in children and adult women than in adult men (Table 9.1).

Table 9.1. Blood lead levels at which no more than 5% of the population will show the indicated intensity of effect

Biochemical effect[a]	Intensity of effect	Population	Blood lead level (μg/l)
ALAD inhibition in red blood cells	> 70% inhibition	adults	300
		children	250–300
ALA in urine	> 10 mg/litre	adults, children	500
FEP in red blood cells	perceptible increase	adult males	300
		adult females	250
		children	200

Source: WHO, 1977.
[a] ALAD = aminolevulinic acid dehydrogenase; ALA = aminolevulinic acid; FEP = free erythrocyte protoporphyrin.

Fig. 9.2. Individual characteristics that modify the effect of environmental factors

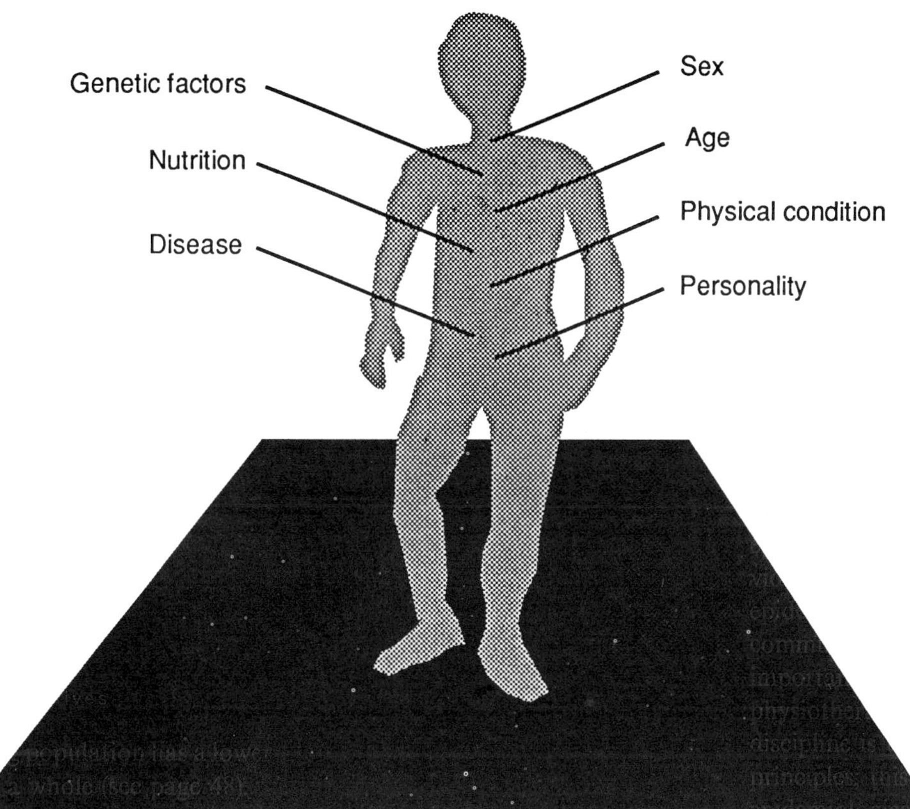

The main emphasis in environmental and occupational epidemiology has been on studies of the causes of disease. Increasing attention is now being given to the evaluation of specific preventive measures to reduce exposure, and of the impact of occupational health services. As exposure to hazardous environmental factors is often the result of some industrial or agricultural activity that brings economic benefit to the community, it may be costly to eliminate them. However, environmental pollution is often costly in itself and may damage agricultural land or industrial property as well as people's health. Epidemiological analyses help public health authorities to find an acceptable balance between health risks and the economic costs of prevention.

Environmental epidemiology will face new challenges in the coming decades with changes in the global environment. Studies will be needed of the potential impact on health of global temperature changes, depletion of the ozone layer, ultraviolet radiation, acid precipitation, and aspects of population dynamics (McMichael, 1991).

Exposure and dose

General concepts

Epidemiological studies on the effects of environmental factors often deal with very specific factors that can be measured quantitatively. The concepts of exposure and dose (see page 79) are therefore particularly important in environmental and occupational epidemiology.

Exposure has two dimensions: level and duration. For environmental factors that cause acute effects more or less immediately after exposure starts, the current exposure level determines whether effects occur (for instance, the "London smog epidemic" of deaths from lung and heart disease, Fig. 9.3).

However, many environmental factors produce effects only after a long period of exposure. This is true of chemicals that accumulate in the body (for instance, cadmium) and hazards that have a cumulative effect (for instance, radiation or noise). For these hazards, the past exposure levels and the exposure duration are more important than the current exposure level. The total exposure (or external

Fig. 9.3. The London smog epidemic, December 1952

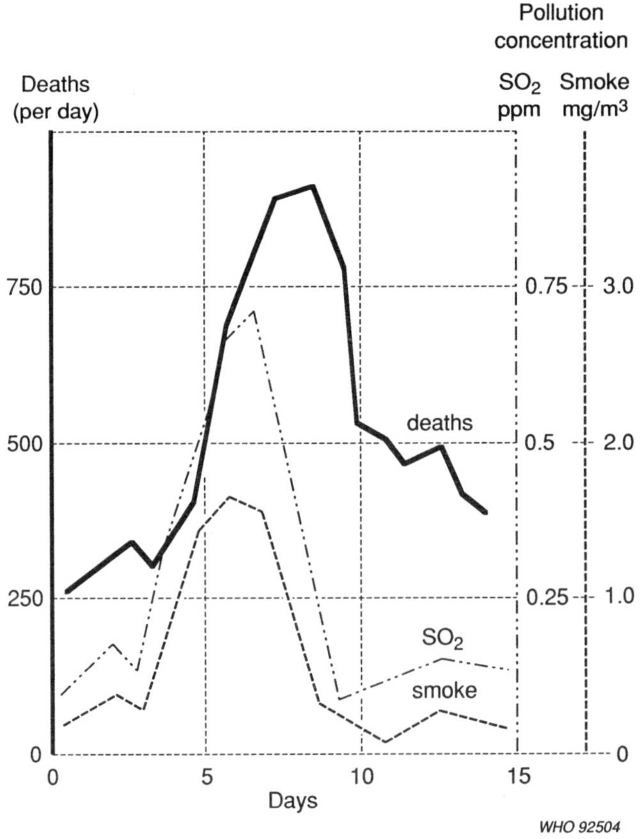

Source: United Kingdom Ministry of Health, 1954.

dose) needs to be estimated. It is often approximated as the product of exposure duration and exposure level.

In epidemiological studies, all kinds of estimates of exposure and dose have been used to quantify the relationship between an environmental factor and the health status of a population. For example, in Fig. 1.1 the exposure is expressed in terms of exposure level only (number of cigarettes smoked per day). Table 5.2 shows the combined effect of duration and exposure level on noise-induced hearing loss. The external dose can also be expressed as one combined measure, as with pack-years for cigarette smoking and fibre-years (or particle-years) for asbestos exposure in the workplace (see Fig. 9.4).

Biological monitoring

If the environmental factor under study is a chemical, the exposure level and dose can sometimes be estimated by measuring the concentration in body fluids or tissues. This approach is called biological monitoring. Blood and urine are most commonly used for biological monitoring, but for certain chemicals other body tissues and fluids may be of particular interest: hair is useful for studies of exposure to methylmercury from fish; nail clippings have been used to study

Fig. 9.4. Relationship between asbestos exposure (particle-years) and relative risk of lung cancer

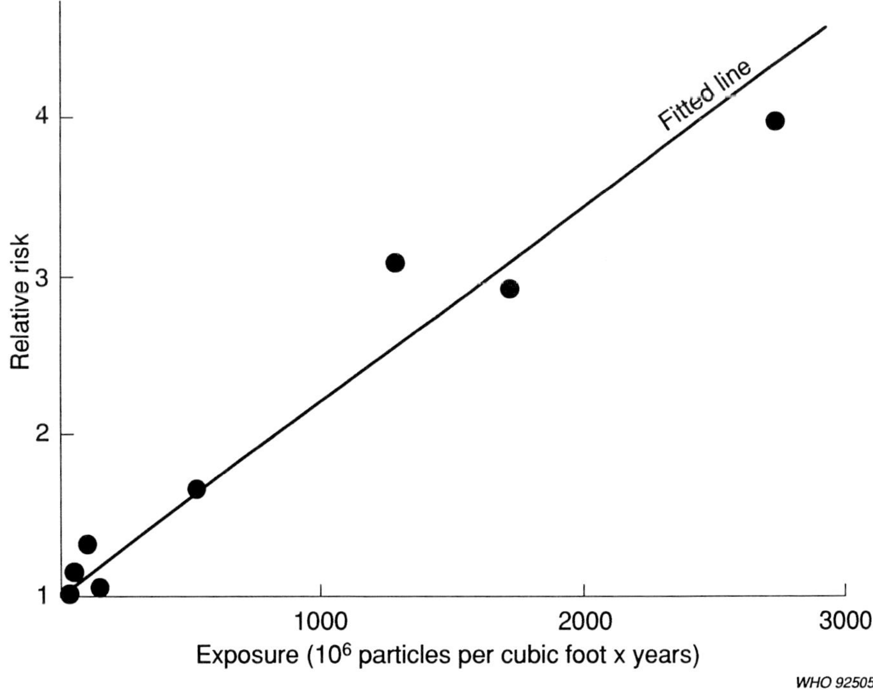

Source: McDonald et al., 1980.

arsenic exposure; analysis of faeces can give an estimate of recent exposure to metals via food; breast milk is a good material for examining exposure to organochlorine pesticides and other chlorinated hydrocarbons such as polychlorinated biphenyls and dioxins; and biopsies of fat, bone, lung, liver and kidney have been used in studies of patients with suspected poisoning.

The interpretation of biological monitoring data requires detailed knowledge of the kinetics and metabolism of chemicals, which includes data on absorption, transport, accumulation and excretion. Because of the rapid excretion of certain chemicals, only the most recent exposure to them can be measured. Sometimes one body tissue or fluid gives an indication of recent exposure and another indicates the total dose. As the chemical would have to be absorbed to reach the biological indicator material, the dose measured in this way is called the absorbed dose or internal dose, as opposed to the external dose estimated from environmental measurements.

Fig. 9.5 shows a rapid increase in blood cadmium in the first months after exposure started, whereas no change in urine cadmium can be detected. On the other hand, after long-term exposure there is a close correlation between urine cadmium and the total dose in the body (Fig. 9.6).

Individual versus group measurements

Individual measurements of exposure vary with time. The frequency of measurements and the method used to estimate the exposure or dose in an epi-

Fig. 9.5. Blood and urine levels of cadmium during the first year of occupational exposure

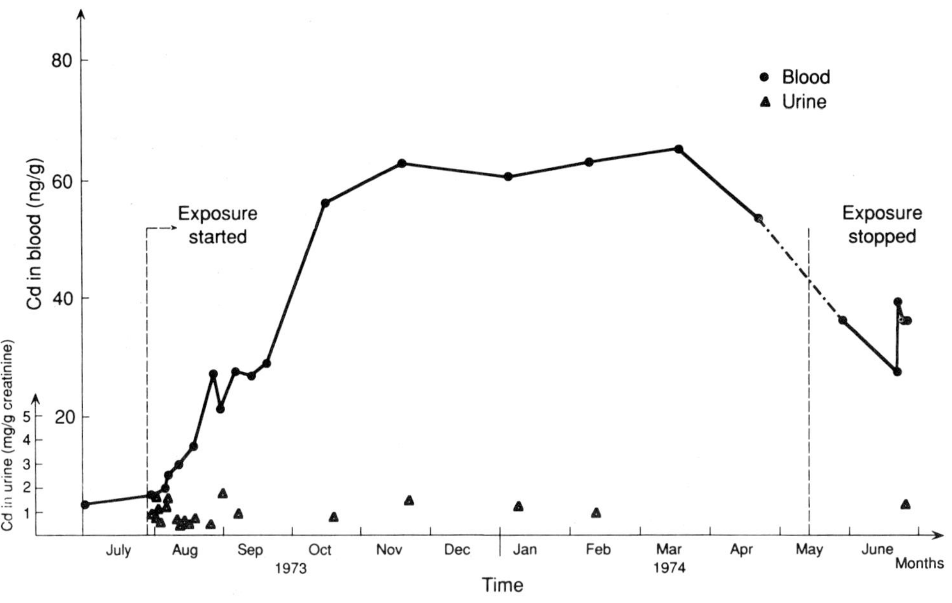

Source: Kjellström & Nordberg, 1978.

Fig. 9.6. Relationship between cadmium dose and urine cadmium

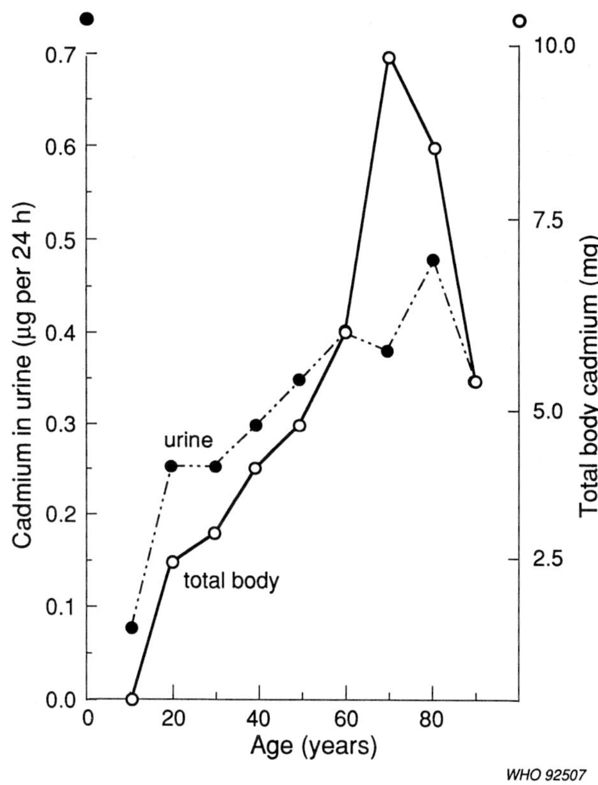

Source: Kjellström, 1977.

demiological study therefore require careful consideration. The estimate used needs to be valid (see Chapter 2) and the measurements need to be accompanied by appropriate quality assurance procedures.

There is also a variation in exposure or dose between individuals. Even people working side-by-side in a factory have different exposure levels because of different work habits or differences in the local distribution of a pollutant. For instance, one machine may leak fumes while another may not. If the exposure or dose is measured by biological monitoring, an additional source of variation is the difference of individual absorption and excretion rates for the chemical. Even people with the same external dose may end up with different internal doses.

One way of presenting individual variations is through distribution curves (Chapter 4). The distributions of individual doses of chemicals are often skewed and conform to a log normal frequency distribution more closely than to a normal distribution. Ideally, the shape of the dose distribution should be tested in every epidemiological study where quantitative dose measurements are carried out. If the distributions are found to be log normal, group comparisons should be carried out with geometric rather than arithmetic means and standard deviations (see page 59).

When presenting the exposure or dose data for groups, arithmetic or geometric means are most commonly used. Another way is to use quantiles or percentiles (Chapter 4). For instance, in assessing whether the dose of lead in a group of children is of concern, the average may be of less interest than the proportion with individual doses above a certain threshold (Fig. 9.7). If a blood lead level of 400 μg/l is the threshold of concern for effects of lead on the brain, then information about the mean level in the group (300 μg/l in 1971) gives no indication of how many children could be affected. It is more informative that 25% of the children had blood lead levels above 400 μg/l in 1971. In 1976 the mean blood lead level had decreased to 200 μg/l and the proportion above 400 μg/l was only 4%.

The same considerations regarding presentation of means or percentiles are important for measurements of effect. There is increasing concern about the effects of environmental chemicals on the intellectual development and behaviour of children. In some studies the intelligence quotient (IQ) has been measured. Differences in the average IQ between groups are often very small (Table 9.2) and the subgroups of special concern consist of children with particularly low IQs. However, a small drop in mean IQ from 107 to 102 can produce a large increase in the proportion with an IQ below 70 (from 0.6% to 2%).

In epidemiological studies of cancer caused by environmental or occupational factors, another way of presenting group dose is sometimes used. This is the dose commitment or population dose, calculated as the sum of individual doses. The

Fig. 9.7. Cumulative distribution of blood lead in black children in New York City, 1971 and 1976

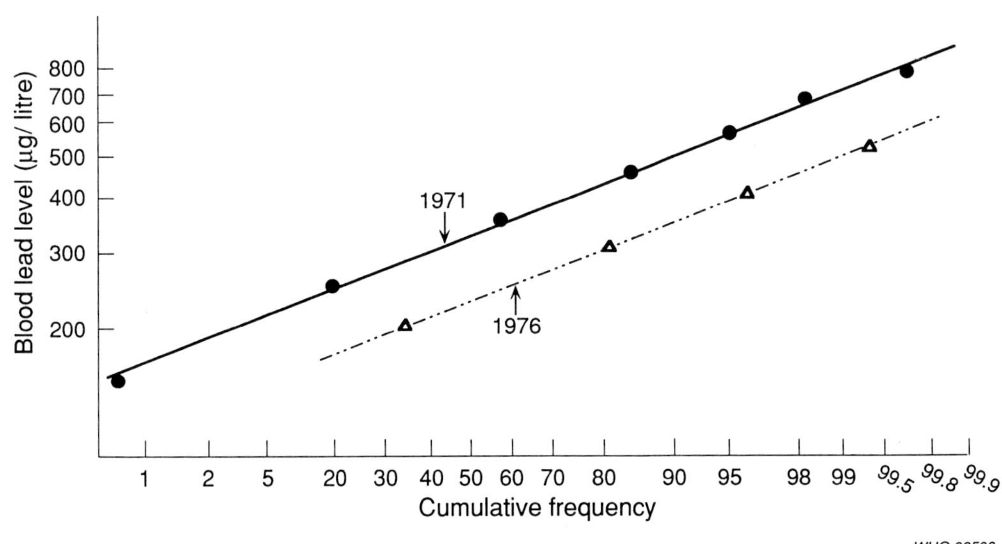

Source: Billick et al., 1979. Reproduced by kind permission of the publisher.

Table 9.2. Full-scale and subtest scores on the Wechsler Intelligence Scale for Children (Revised) (WISC-R) for subjects with high and low lead levels in teeth

WISC-R	Low lead (< 10 mg/kg) (mean)	High lead (> 20 mg/kg) (mean)	*P* value (one-sided)
Full-scale IQ	106.6	102.1	0.03
Verbal IQ	103.9	99.3	0.03
Information	10.5	9.4	0.04
Vocabulary	11.0	10.0	0.05
Digit span	10.6	9.3	0.02
Arithmetic	10.4	10.1	0.49
Comprehension	11.0	10.2	0.08
Similarities	10.8	10.3	0.36
Performance IQ	108.7	104.9	0.08
Picture completion	12.2	11.3	0.03
Picture arrangement	11.3	10.8	0.38
Block design	11.0	10.3	0.15
Object assembly	10.9	10.6	0.54
Coding	11.0	10.9	0.90
Mazes	10.6	10.1	0.37

Source: Needleman et al., 1979. Reproduced by kind permission of the publisher.

theory is that this total population dose is what determines the number of cancers that will occur. For radiation, a dose commitment of 50 sievert (Sv) is expected to cause one fatal cancer. Whether the dose commitment refers to 100 people each with a dose of 0.5 Sv or 10 000 people each with a dose of 5 mSv, the result is one case of fatal cancer. This calculation is based on the fundamental assumptions that there is no threshold individual dose below which the cancer risk is zero and that the cancer risk increases linearly with dose.

Dose–effect relationships

For many environmental factors, effects range from subtle physiological or biochemical changes to severe illness or death, as explained in Chapter 2. Usually, the higher the dose, the more severe or intense is the effect. This relationship between dose and severity of effect is called the dose–effect relationship (Fig. 9.8), which can be established for an individual or a group (the average dose at which each effect occurs). Not all individuals react in the same way to a given environmental exposure, so the dose–effect relationship for an individual differs from the group value.

The dose–effect relationship provides valuable information for the planning of epidemiological studies. Some effects may be easier to measure than others, and some may be of particular significance for public health. The dose–effect relationship helps the investigator to choose an appropriate effect to study.

Fig. 9.8. Dose–effect relationship

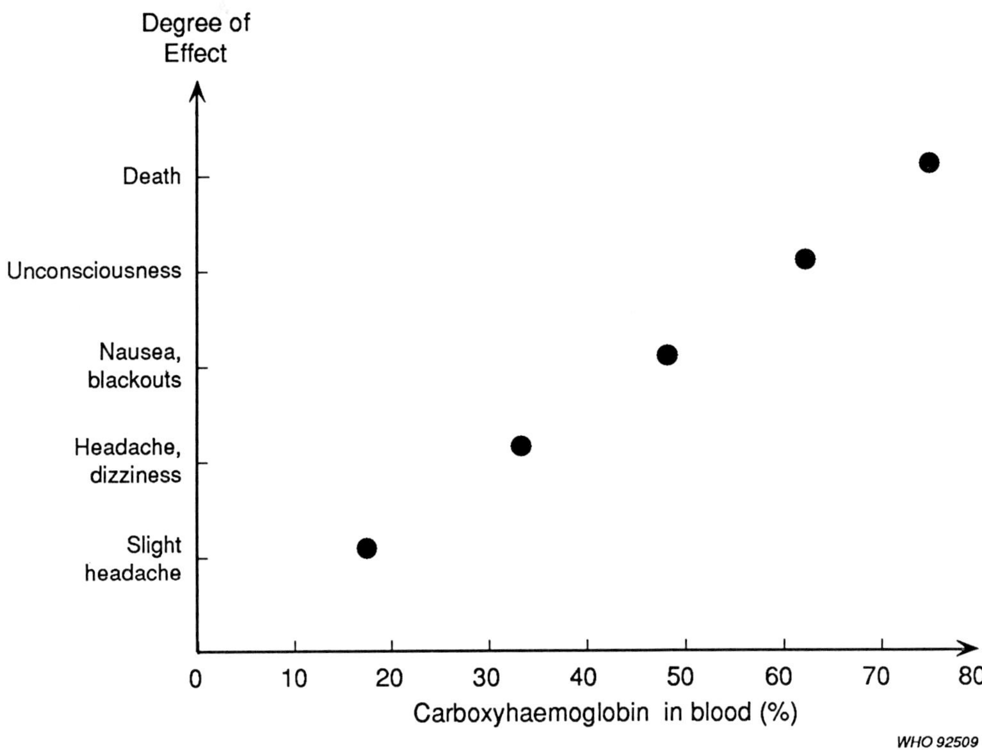

In the process of establishing safety standards, the dose–effect relationship also gives useful information on effects that must be prevented and on those that may be used for screening purposes. If a safety standard is set at a level where the less severe effects are prevented, the more severe effects are also likely to be prevented because they occur at higher doses.

Dose–response relationships

Response is defined in epidemiology as the proportion of an exposed group that develops a specific effect. Fig. 9.9 shows the dose–response relationship most commonly seen in epidemiological studies.

At low doses almost nobody suffers the effect and at a high level almost everybody does so. This reflects the variation in individual sensitivity to the factor studied. The S-shaped curve in Fig. 9.9 is of the type expected if individual sensitivity follows a normal distribution. Many examples of dose–response relationships with this shape have been found in environmental and occupational epidemiology studies.

The dose–response phenomenon can in some cases be approximated to a straight-line relationship, particularly when only a narrow range of low responses is involved. This approach has been used, for instance, to study the relationship between cancer risk and radiation dose or asbestos dose (Fig. 9.4).

Fig. 9.9. Dose–response relationship

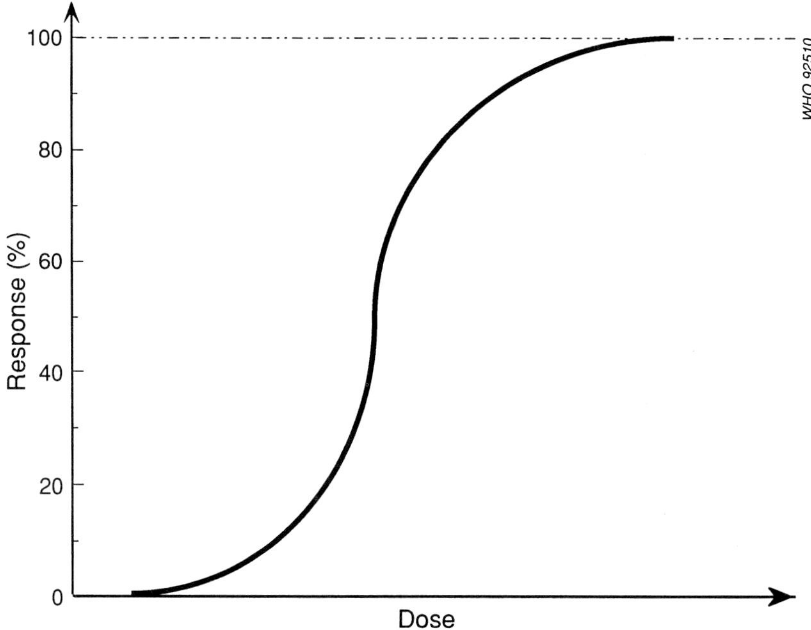

The dose–response relationship can be modified by factors such as age. This has been found, for instance, for hearing loss caused by loud noise (WHO, 1980a), one of the most common health effects in the workplace.

Risk assessment and risk management

In recent years, increased attention has been given to the use of epidemiological principles to estimate the potential health risks of industrial or agricultural development projects, both before they are implemented and while they are in operation. Environmental impact assessment (predictive analysis) and environmental audit (analysis of the existing situation) have become legal requirements in many countries. The health component of these activities is one of the important applications of risk assessment. Such assessment is also used to predict potential health problems in the use of new chemicals or technologies. The term risk management is applied to the planning and implementation of actions to reduce or eliminate the health risk (WHO, 1989c).

The first step in a risk assessment is to identify which environmental health hazard may be created by the technology or project under study. Are there chemical hazards? If so, which specific chemicals are involved? Are there biological hazards? etc. (see Fig. 9.1). The next step involves an analysis of the type of health effect that each hazard may cause (hazard assessment). The information can be collected by reviewing the scientific literature for each hazard or referring to available reliable hazard assessments, such as the

Environmental Health Criteria Series published by WHO, or the Monograph Series published by the International Agency for Research on Cancer (IARC), and, if necessary, complementing this by epidemiological studies of people exposed to the hazards in question.

The third step is to measure or estimate the actual exposure levels for the people potentially affected, including the general population and the workforce. The human exposure assessment should take into account environmental monitoring, biological monitoring, and relevant information about history of exposure and changes over time. As a fourth step, the exposure data for subgroups of the exposed population are combined with the dose–effect and dose–response relationships for each hazard to calculate the likely health risk in this population. Epidemiological studies can also be used to measure directly the health risk. The risk could be presented as potential increase in relative risk of certain health effects or the calculated increase in the number of cases of certain diseases or symptoms.

Risk management involves three main steps. First, estimates of health risk need to be evaluated in relation to a predetermined "acceptable risk" or in relation to other health risks in the same community. Maximum exposure limits, public health targets, or other policy instruments for health protection are often used in this process. The fundamental question is: is it necessary to take preventive action because the estimated health risk is too high?

If it is decided that preventive action is needed, the next step in risk management is to reduce exposure. This may involve changing the processes to eliminate certain hazards, installing equipment to control pollution, resiting proposed hazardous projects, etc.

Finally, risk management also involves the monitoring of exposure and health risks after the selected controls have been put into place. It is important to ensure that the intended protection is achieved and that any additional protective measures are taken without delay. In this phase of risk management, human exposure assessments and epidemiological surveys play an important role.

Special features of environmental and occupational epidemiology

The uses of epidemiology in these fields include all those listed in Chapter 1, i.e. etiology, natural history, the description of the health status of a population, and the evaluation of interventions and health services. One special feature of many etiological studies in occupational epidemiology is the use of company or trade union records to identify individuals with past exposure to a specific hazard or type of work. With the help of such records, retrospective cohort studies can be carried out. A number of associations between occupational hazards and health effects have been identified in this way.

Dose–effect and dose–response relationships are of particular importance in environmental and occupational epidemiology because they provide the foundation for the setting of safety standards. The dose–effect relationship can be used to decide which effect it is most important to prevent. If a decision is then made concerning an acceptable response level the dose–response relationship gives the maximum dose that would be acceptable. WHO has developed a series of air quality guidelines (WHO, 1987d) and health-based maximum occupational exposure limits (WHO, 1980c) using this approach. In response to the accident at the Chernobyl nuclear power station, guidelines were also developed for radioactive contamination of food (WHO, 1988b). For many environmental factors the available data are insufficient to permit a standard to be set with any accuracy, and informed guessing or practical experience becomes the basis of the safety standard. Further epidemiological studies in this field are needed to provide more information on dose–response relationships.

As mentioned earlier, occupational epidemiology studies often include only men who are physically fit. The exposed group of workers thus has a lower overall mortality rate than the corresponding age group in the general population. The lower mortality has been called the healthy worker effect (McMichael, 1976), which needs to be taken into account whenever the mortality rate in a group of workers is compared with the rate in the general population. Often the rates among healthy workers are 70–90% of those in the general population. The

Fig. 9.10. Relationship between driving speed, seat-belt use, and frequency of injury in motor car drivers involved in collisions

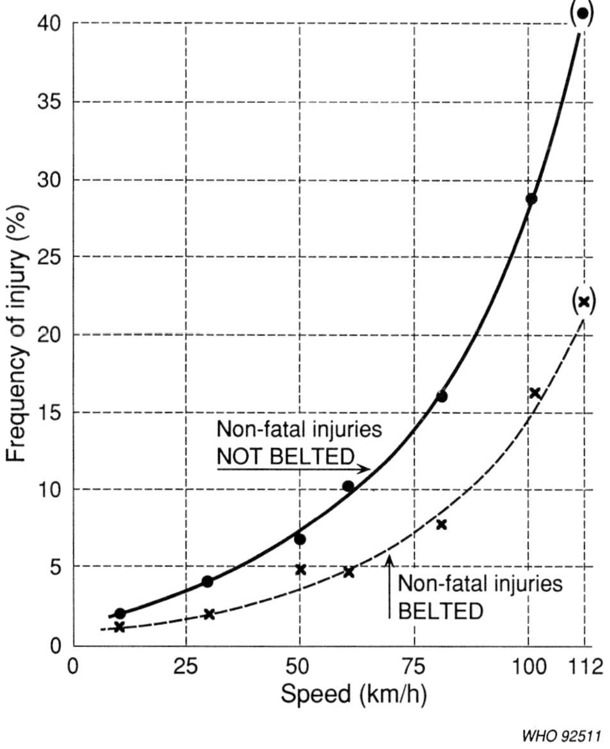

Source: Bohlin, 1967. Reproduced by kind permission of the publisher.

difference arises because of the presence of unhealthy and disabled people in the non-working population who usually have higher mortality rates.

One special type of epidemiological analysis that plays an important role in environmental and occupational health is accident and injury epidemiology. Traffic accident injuries are on the increase in many countries and, being a major cause of death and illness among young people, they have a great impact on public health.

Similarly, accidental injuries are among the most important types of ill health caused by factors in the workplace. The environmental factors associated with these injuries are often more difficult to identify and quantify than those causing, for instance, chemical poisoning. In addition, the term "accident" gives the impression of some random occurrence leading to injury, a notion that discourages systematic epidemiological studies of the factors causing accidental or unintentional injuries.

Exposure and dose in accident epidemiology studies often have to be measured indirectly. Fig. 9.10 shows the relationship between driving speed (dose) and frequency of injury (response) for drivers in traffic accidents; this is valuable information for decisions regarding two different preventive approaches: speed reduction and the use of seat-belts.

Study questions

9.1 (a) For which effects is there a difference in susceptibility to lead between the groups in Table 9.1?

(b) Which group is most susceptible?

9.2 (a) What is the result of the increasing external dose shown in Fig. 9.4?

(b) Why are asbestos doses often calculated as particle–years or fibre–years?

9.3 (a) The blood level of cadmium increases after the start of exposure and reaches a plateau after about three months (Fig. 9.5). What is the implication for the use of blood cadmium as a measure of exposure in a cross-sectional study of workers?

(b) Six months after a new production process is introduced in a copper smelter, a suspicion of cadmium pollution is raised. How can biological monitoring of residents in the potentially polluted area help to distinguish between a new cadmium pollution problem and one that has existed for many years (see Fig. 9.5 and 9.6)?

9.4 You are a public health official in a medium-sized city with a number of large industrial enterprises. The workers in these enterprises are provided with medical care through a uniform insurance system, which means that all current and retired workers are likely to get health care from the same hospital. A hospital doctor calls you and expresses concern about the large number of lung cancers among the workers. How would you design an initial study to investigate potential associations between occupational exposures and increased risk of lung cancer?

9.5 How could an epidemiological analysis of the London smog epidemic of deaths due to heart and lung disease in 1952 (Fig. 9.3) ascertain that the epidemic was in fact due to smog?

9.6 What is meant by the healthy worker effect and how can it introduce bias in occupational epidemiology studies?

Chapter 10
Epidemiology, health services and health policy

Health care planning and evaluation

The systematic use of epidemiological principles and methods for the planning and evaluation of health services is a relatively new development. From the assessment of the value of specific treatments it is a short step to the assessment of more general aspects of health services. The ultimate goal is to develop a rational process for setting priorities and allocating scarce health care resources. Because of the limited resources available for health care in all countries, choices have to be made between alternative strategies for improving health.

Health service planning is a process of identifying key objectives and choosing among alternative means of achieving them. Evaluation is the process of determining, as systematically and objectively as possible, the relevance, effectiveness, efficiency and impact of activities with respect to the agreed goals.

In this chapter the process of planning for and evaluating a health care intervention directed towards a specific disease will be illustrated. The same process should be adopted in broader interventions, such as the development of a national care programme for the elderly or of a new approach to the delivery of primary health care in rural areas.

In all these activities, epidemiologists work alongside a variety of other specialists who together provide the community and its decision-makers with information so that policy choices can be made on the basis of a reasonable knowledge of the likely outcomes and costs.

The planning cycle

Fig. 10.1 shows the steps involved in the health care planning process and provides a useful framework for ensuring that the information required by policy-makers is identified. Usually, only part of the information needed for making decisions is available and it always has to be critically assessed. If the information is insufficient, new data have to be collected to ensure that policy choices can be made in a rational manner.

The process is cyclical and repetitive and the steps are:

(1) measurement or assessment of the burden of illness;

(2) identification of the causes of illness;

(3) measurement of the effectiveness of different community interventions;

(4) assessment of their efficiency in terms of resources used;

Fig. 10.1. The health care planning cycle

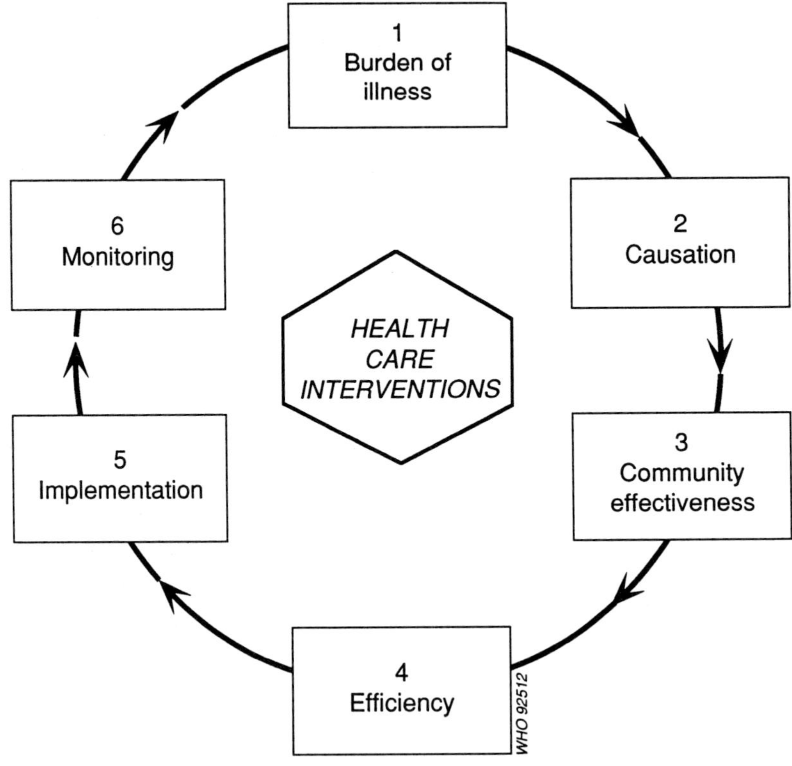

Source: Tugwell et al., 1985. Reproduced by kind permission of the publisher.

(5) implementation of interventions;

(6) monitoring of activities;

(7) reassessment of the burden of illness to determine whether it has been altered.

Epidemiology is involved at all stages of planning. The cyclical nature of the process indicates the importance of monitoring and evaluation to determine whether the interventions have had the desired effects. The process is repetitive because each cycle of intervention usually has only a small impact on the burden of illness, and repeated intervention is required.

Burden of illness

Measurement of the overall health status of the community (see Chapter 2) is the first step in the planning process. The measurements can include prevalence rates, incidence rates, different measures of mortality, and the number of cases of different diseases. The process of measuring the burden of illness must include indicators that fully assess the effects of disease on society. Mortality data reflect only one aspect of health and are of limited value in respect of conditions that are rarely fatal. Measures of morbidity reflect another important aspect of the burden of illness. In addition, increasing attention is being given to measuring the consequences of disease, i.e. impairment, disability and handicap (see page 28). The burden of illness, in terms of the number of cases created by a particular environmental factor, is called its public health impact.

Increasing attention is being given to the development of improved epidemiological techniques for assessing health problems and evaluating health programmes in developing countries. Rapid epidemiological assessment is now a defined field of epidemiological research, and includes small-area survey and sampling methods, surveillance methods, screening and individual risk assessment, community indicators of risk and health status, and case–control methods for evaluation (Smith, 1989).

Summary measurements of the burden of illness must be accurate and simple to interpret; an important development is the introduction of measures that include both mortality and quality-of-life considerations. One such measure, called quality-adjusted life years, is becoming popular in cost–effectiveness and cost–benefit analyses. Another, termed life expectancy free from disability or healthy life expectancy, has been developed mainly by demographers and is increasingly being used in industrialized countries (Robine, 1989). Many assumptions are involved in the use of these sophisticated indices and caution is required in their interpretation, but they offer the prospect of rationalizing the choice of options in health services.

The evaluation of health services must start with knowledge about the burden of illness and its long-term effects, and consequently about the *need* and *demand* for health services in the population. The need is determined by both value judgements and by the ability of health services to influence the particular problems. Needs may or may not be met by health services. If a need is not met, the lack may or may not be perceived. Demand, on the other hand, refers to the population's willingness and ability to seek, use and, in some settings, pay for health services. Demand for a service may arise from patients or doctors and may be closely related to or in excess of need. Not all demand can be met by health services. Occasionally, unnecessary demands are met, as with superfluous investigations or operations.

The measurement of need requires a defined population base, and the relationship of need to demand can only be established by epidemiological studies. In the USA, for example, community surveys of blood pressure have established the frequency of undiagnosed hypertension (unmet need) and how this has fallen since the 1970s as a result of blood pressure control programmes (Table 10.1).

Causation

Once the burden of illness in the community has been measured, it is necessary to try to identify the major preventable causes of disease so that intervention strategies can be developed. Wherever possible, interventions should have the prevention of disease as their primary focus but, of course, this is not always possible.

Table 10.1. Percentage of adult population (18–74 years) with undiagnosed hypertension, by race and time, in the USA

Race	1971–74	1976–80
White	11.2	7.6
Black	17.1	6.9

Source: Drizd et al., 1986.

The role of epidemiology in identifying causal factors is discussed more fully in Chapter 5.

Measuring effectiveness of different interventions

The need for measurement of the effectiveness of interventions is illustrated in Table 10.2, which indicates how the length of hospital stay for patients with acute myocardial infarction has decreased since the 1950s. The main questions raised by these data are: "Are patients arriving sooner after the initial symptoms?", "Is treatment becoming more effective?", "What is the appropriate length of stay?", and "Are some patients being harmed by premature discharge?" These questions can best be addressed through well-designed randomized controlled trials (see page 42).

The most important information that should be available to facilitate decision-making on resource allocation concerns the relationships between health intervention programmes and changes in health status. Such relationships can be characterized in both qualitative and quantitative terms. The structure of a health service organization and the process of health care, i.e. the activities of health personnel, can be described. However, qualitative approaches, although important, provide only limited information on the ultimate success or otherwise of a health service. Quantitative data need to be analysed as well. Effectiveness is measured in terms of percentage reduction in morbidity or mortality as a result of a specific intervention.

Table 10.2. Variation in length of hospital stay for patients with uncomplicated acute myocardial infarction

Time	Length of stay
1950s	4–8 weeks
1960s	3 weeks
1970	2 weeks
1980	7–10 days
1988	4–5 days

Source: Curfman, 1988.

The effectiveness of interventions in the community is determined by many factors, including the following.

- How well an intervention works under ideal conditions, i.e. when great attention is given to diagnosis and long-term management and follow-up (efficacy; see page 113). This situation is usually only found in randomized controlled trials; if the intervention does not work under these conditions, it is unlikely to work in the community. Well-conducted randomized controlled trials have shown, for example, that the treatment of mild hypertension reduces rates of fatal and nonfatal stroke by about 40%. However, the effectiveness of antihypertensive treatment in community application is less pronounced (Bonita & Beaglehole, 1989) because some people who are offered treatment do not follow the regimen.
- The ability to screen for and diagnose the disease accurately (see Chapter 6); both the health care provider and the consumer must be compliant with the necessary actions.
- The appropriate use of the intervention by all who could benefit; this means that the intervention has to be both available and acceptable to the community.

Efficiency

Efficiency is a measure of the relationship between the results achieved and the effort expended in terms of money, resources and time. It provides the basis for the optimal use of resources and involves the complex interrelationship of costs and effectiveness of an intervention. This is an area where epidemiology and health economics are applied together.

There are two main approaches to the assessment of efficiency. *Cost–effectiveness analysis*, looks at the ratio of financial expenditure and effectiveness: dollars per life-year gained, dollars per case prevented, dollars per quality-adjusted life-year gained, and so on. In *cost–benefit analysis*, both the numerator and denominator are expressed in monetary terms. This means that health benefits (for example, lives saved) must be measured and given a monetary value. If the cost–benefit analysis shows that economic benefits of the programme are greater than the costs, the programme should be seriously considered.

Cost–effectiveness analysis is easier to perform than cost–benefit analysis, since the measure of effectiveness does not need to be given a monetary value. Table 10.3 summarizes the estimated costs in the United Kingdom for each extra quality-adjusted life-year gained as a result of various procedures.

Although these estimates are based on approximate information and many assumptions, they are useful to policy-makers who have to set priorities. The measurement of efficiency requires many assumptions and it should be used very cautiously; it is not value-free and can serve only as a general guideline.

In the developing world there is increasing interest in the economic aspects of proposed health programmes. However, only a few studies have carried out

Table 10.3. Estimated cost of each extra quality-adjusted life year (QALY) gained as a result of selected procedures

Procedure	Cost per QALY gained (pounds sterling)
Aortic valve replacement	900
Pacemaker	700
Heart transplant	5 000
Kidney transplant	3 000
Hospital haemodialysis	14 000
Home haemodialysis	11 000
Hip replacement	750

Source: Williams, 1985. Reproduced by kind permission of the publisher.

formal economic assessment. The principles of such studies and their problems have been reviewed by Mills (1985).

Implementation

The fifth stage in the planning process begins with decisions on specific interventions and takes into account the problems likely to be faced in and by the community. For example, if screening for breast cancer by mammography is planned, it is important to ensure that the necessary equipment and personnel are available. This stage involves the setting of specific quantified targets, e.g. "to reduce the frequency of smoking in young women from 30% to 20% over a five-year period". This type of target-setting is essential for assessing the success of an intervention.

Monitoring

Monitoring is the continuous follow-up of activities to ensure that they are proceeding according to plan. Monitoring must be directed to requirements of specific programmes, the success of which may be measured in a variety of ways using short-, intermediate- and long-term criteria.

For a community hypertension programme, monitoring could include the regular assessment of:

- personnel training;
- the availability and accuracy of sphygmomanometers (structural);
- the appropriateness of case-finding and management procedures (process evaluation);
- the effect on blood-pressure levels in treated patients (outcome evaluation).

Reassessment of the burden of illness

Reassessment is the final step in the health care planning process (Table 10.4) and the first step in the next cycle of activity (Fig. 10.1). Reasssessment requires a

Table 10.4. Health care planning: the case of hypertension

Burden	Population surveys of blood pressure and control of hypertension
Etiology	Ecological studies (salt and blood pressure) Observational studies (weight and blood pressure) Experimental studies (weight reduction)
Community effectiveness	Randomized controlled trials Evaluation of screening programmes Studies of compliance
Efficiency	Cost–effectiveness studies
Implementation	National control programmes for high blood pressure
Monitoring	Assessment of personnel and equipment Effect on quality of life
Reassessment	Remeasurement of population blood pressure levels

repeat measurement of the burden of illness in the population by, for example, repeated surveys of population blood pressure levels.

Epidemiology, public policy and health policy

Public policy is the sum of the decisions that shape society. It provides a framework for the development of, for example, industrial and agricultural production, corporate management, and health services. It outlines the range of options from which organizations and individuals make their choices, and thus directly influences the environment and patterns of living. Public policy is a major determinant of the health of the population. Health policy usually refers specifically to medical care issues, but health is influenced by a broad range of policy decisions, not just those in the medical or health field. A true health policy should therefore provide a framework for health-promoting actions in the general economy of a community as well as in agriculture, industry, labour, energy, transport and education.

If epidemiology is to be successful in leading to the prevention and control of diseases, epidemiological research results must influence public policy, including health policy. To date, epidemiology has not fulfilled its potential in this respect, and there are only a few areas in which epidemiological research has been fully applied. However, the importance of epidemiology in policy-making is increasingly recognized.

The influence of epidemiology is usually mediated by public opinion. Policy-makers in many countries often respond to public opinion rather than leading it. The growth in media attention given to epidemiological research has increased public awareness of the subject. Epidemiology is often an important factor influencing public policy but is rarely the only one doing so.

A major difficulty in applying epidemiology to public policy is the necessity for making judgements about the cause of a disease and decisions on what to do about it when the evidence is incomplete. Some epidemiologists believe their role should be limited to epidemiological research, while others consider they should be directly involved in the application of the results to public policy, a difference reflecting personal, social and cultural preferences. If a health issue is controversial, the involvement of epidemiologists in the public policy arena may lead to criticisms of bias or one-sidedness.

In the application of epidemiology to public policy in a given country, difficult decisions have to be made about the relevance of research done in other countries since it is usually impossible, and probably unnecessary, for major studies to be repeated. However, some local evidence is usually required before a strong case can be made for a policy change or costly interventions.

In 1986 the Ottawa Charter for Health Promotion made it clear that health is influenced by a wide range of policy decisions. Health policy is not simply the responsibility of health departments. Policy decisions by a wide range of agencies, both governmental and nongovernmental, have a significant impact on health. A concern for health and equity is needed in all areas of public policy. Agricultural policies influence the availability, price and quality of meat and dairy products; advertising and fiscal policies influence the price and availability of cigarettes; transport policies influence the extent of urban air pollution and the risk of traffic accidents.

This broad social policy approach, although often described in rather vague terms, contrasts with much health policy, which, although firmly grounded on the results of epidemiological research, has been directed almost exclusively towards individuals or groups and has paid little attention to the potential range of options.

In many countries, WHO's health-for-all strategy provides the basis for health policy. A central focus of this strategy is the setting of health goals and targets. The approach varies but in each country this is done in accordance with epidemiological knowledge.

In the USA an elaborate and comprehensive list of 226 health objectives was drawn up in 1980 with a target date of 1990. Progress was reviewed midway through the decade, at which time approximately half of the objectives had either been achieved or were on schedule to be achieved by 1990 (McGinnis, 1990; United States Department of Health and Human Services, 1986). In New Zealand, a more modest set of health goals and targets has been established (New Zealand Department of Health, 1989).

Healthy public policy in practice

The goal of a healthy public policy is health promotion, i.e. to enable people to increase control over and to improve their health. It is also essential to create supportive environments, strengthen community action, develop personal skills and reorient health services (Fig. 10.2).

The time-scale for the application of epidemiological research to policy varies; especially with chronic diseases, it can be measured in decades rather than years.

Fig. 10.2. Healthy public policy

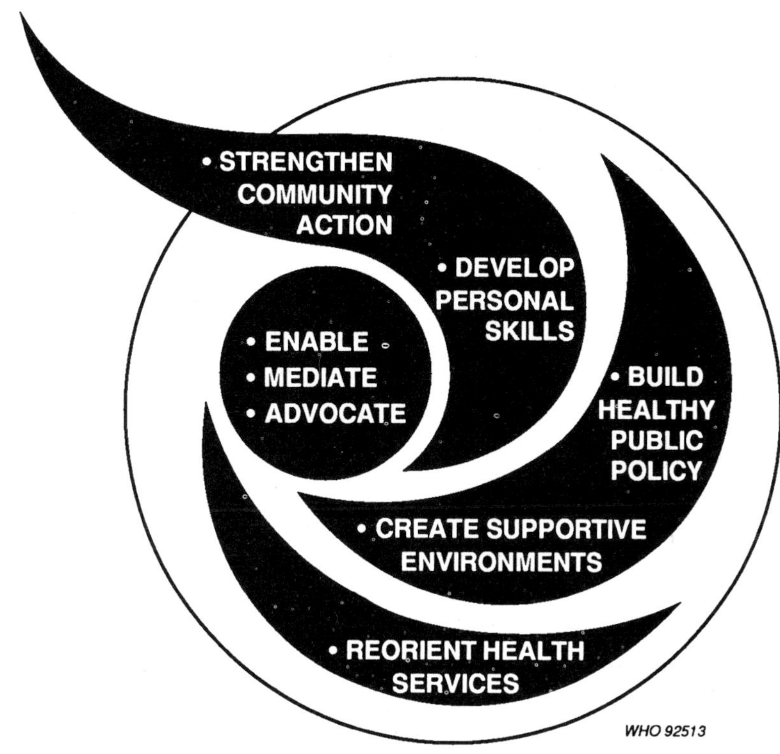

Source: Ottawa Charter for Health Promotion, 1986.

Table 10.5 outlines the findings of research on coronary heart disease and the resulting policy decisions in the USA. The steps in the evolution of public policy in this instance parallel the health care planning process discussed earlier in this chapter.

By the early 1950s, the public health significance of coronary heart disease was appreciated, although little was known about the risk factors. The link between serum cholesterol and coronary heart disease was suspected on the basis of animal experiments even before the initiation of major epidemiological studies. Early pathological investigations had shown that cholesterol was a major component of atherosclerotic lesions in humans. Influential international studies began to explore the role of dietary fat in the 1950s, and major cohort studies were undertaken. By the end of the 1950s observational evidence was accumulating on the importance of elevated serum cholesterol, hypertension and smoking as the major risk factors for coronary heart disease.

The observational studies were complemented in the 1960s by the first phase of trials testing the effect of attempts to alter intake of dietary fat on rates of coronary heart disease. Many of these trials were flawed and individually produced no convincing effects, although the trends were consistent. It was soon recognized that definitive trials of dietary factors and coronary heart disease

Table 10.5. Development of healthy public policy with respect to coronary heart disease, USA

Time	Event
1940–1950s	Community burden of coronary heart disease recognized
1950–1960s	Epidemiological evidence accumulates on the importance of major risk factors
1960–1980s	Experimental studies of increasing sophistication are conducted
1960s onwards	Official statements (for example, the American Heart Association) on the significance of risk factors and the importance of prevention
1972 onwards	National High Blood Pressure Education Programme
1985	National Consensus Development Conference on Lipids and Coronary Heart Disease
1986	National High Blood Cholesterol Programme

Source: Syme & Guralnik, 1987.

were impracticable and attention turned to the effect of cholesterol-lowering drugs. A turning point came with the result of a trial in the USA in the 1980s (Lipid Research Clinics Program, 1984).

From a policy perspective, many official pronouncements were made, beginning in 1960 with the first statement of the American Heart Association. In 1985 the National Consensus Development Conference in the USA signalled an increased emphasis on the prevention of coronary heart disease, in particular through attempts to lower cholesterol levels in both high-risk people and the population at large. Elements of this programme include a national education campaign on high cholesterol levels, a laboratory standardization programme, and continued efforts to lower cholesterol levels through strategies aimed at both the population and high-risk groups.

As indicated in Table 10.5, it has taken over 30 years for comprehensive prevention and control policies for coronary heart disease to be introduced. However, the emphasis of public policy on coronary heart disease still lies in attempts to influence individual behaviour, both for members of the health professions and for the public. Relatively little attention has been directed towards long-term community-based prevention programmes and even less to facilitating healthy dietary habits and discouraging smoking at population level. It must be recognized that coronary heart disease is the first major noncommunicable disease to receive such close attention from both researchers and policy-makers. It is possible that more rapid action will be taken to control other major noncommunicable diseases on the basis of the experience gained.

For communicable diseases, action has often been more swift. AIDS was first described in 1981 and within five years policies to limit its spread were being pursued in several countries; for example, legislation to allow the distribution of sterile needles to drug addicts was passed in the Netherlands in 1986 and restrictions on the advertising of condoms were lifted in several countries in the mid-1980s. However, even with AIDS, action has been perceived by many people as proceeding too slowly (Schilts, 1988).

Study questions

10.1 Outline the steps of the health care planning cycle with reference to the problem of falls in the elderly.

10.2 Apply the principles of the Ottawa Charter for Health Promotion to the development of healthy public policy regarding cigarette smoking.

Chapter 11
Continuing your education in epidemiology

Introduction

If the preceding chapters have been successful they will have encouraged you to develop further your epidemiological knowledge and skills. There are several ways in which this can be done:

- by learning more about specific diseases;
- by critically reading the literature on epidemiological investigations;
- by designing and executing small-scale epidemiological projects such as are often included in course work for health professionals;
- by advanced reading in epidemiology, using textbooks, monographs and journals;
- by taking further courses in epidemiology.

Epidemiological knowledge about specific diseases

All health practitioners, including medical practitioners, public health managers, environmental health officers, health researchers, and district health practitioners need to have specific knowledge about a number of health problems and diseases. Epidemiological knowledge is essential, although the extent and type of information required vary with the duties of the practitioners.

Table 11.1 lists the basic items of epidemiological information about a specific disease which would be required to give a full picture. For some diseases additional information would be needed; in most cases it would be obtainable in standard textbooks.

Epidemiological knowledge must be complemented by knowledge about the pathology, clinical practice, pharmacology, rehabilitation and economic impact of the disease. Information about the chemistry, engineering or sanitation aspects of prevention may also be needed in accordance with the responsibilities of specific professions.

Critical reading of published reports

Keeping informed and up to date, even in a narrow specialist field, is a major problem because of the huge quantity of material, varying widely in quality, that is published.

It is therefore necessary to read the medical and health literature critically, so as to be able to make independent judgements of the reliability of information, the

Table 11.1. Basic epidemiological information about a disease

Natural history in the individual:
- development with age (cohort basis)
- early indicators (for screening)
- impact of different treatments
- possibility of cure
- needs for care
- social impact

Etiology:
- specific causal factors
- other risk factors

Development in the community:
- time trends
- variations with age (cross-sectional basis)

Differences in occurrence:
- sex
- ethnic group
- social class
- occupation
- geographical area

Possibilities for prevention:
- specific actions against causal factors
- general actions against other risk factors
- impact of medical services
- impact of health policy

validity of conclusions, and the interpretation of results. A systematic approach and much practice are required if this is to be achieved.

The McMaster system of critical reading categorizes clinical papers into four broad types:

- natural history of disease;
- causes of disease;
- benefits of therapy;
- value of diagnostic tests.

The details of this system have been given by Sackett et al. (1985). It is important for the reader to develop his or her own system of critical reading. With practice it becomes easier to judge the quality of articles. The following questions should be considered when evaluating an article in accordance with the McMaster system.

- *What is the research question?*

The first step for the reader is to determine the objectives of the study, i.e. the question or questions being addressed or the hypothesis being tested. The summary or abstract helps to determine whether the paper is of interest and relevant to the situation in which the reader is working, i.e. whether the patients or subjects are similar to those seen locally. The major question to be considered when reading the abstract is: "If the reported results are true, is the information useful?" If the answer is in the negative, no further reading is necessary. If, on the other hand, the results might be of interest, one has to determine whether they are valid. Attention shifts to determining their accuracy; this requires that the methods be studied critically.

- *What is the population about which the research question is being asked?*
  - Who is included and who is excluded?
  - Are the subjects a sample of the target population? If not, why?
  - How has the sample been selected?
  - Is there evidence of random selection, as opposed to systematic selection or self-selection by volunteers?
  - What possible sources of bias are there in the selection?
  - How might the selection process affect the results?
  - Is the sample large enough to answer the question being addressed?

Separate approaches are required when determining the next step, depending on whether the research presented is an experiment comparing treatments or a survey aimed at observing and estimating quantities or relationships.

For an experiment the following questions are relevant:

- How were subjects assigned to treatments: randomly or in some other way?
- What control groups were included (placebo, untreated controls, both or neither)?
- How were the treatments compared? Was the outcome or response objectively measured?
- Was any chemical analysis or other measurement supported by quality assurance procedures?

For a survey the following questions are appropriate:

- Was the data collection process adequate (including questionnaire design and pre-testing)?
- What techniques were used to handle nonresponse and/or incomplete data?
- What possible sources of bias are evident?
- Was any chemical analysis or other measurement supported by quality assurance procedures?

- *How are the data presented?*
  - Are there sufficient clear graphs and/or tables? Are the numbers consistent? Is the entire sample accounted for?
  - Are standard deviations presented with means, confidence intervals, regression coefficients or other statistics, as well as the raw data?

- Is the sample adequately described in terms of variables related to the question being posed?
- Is there sufficient evidence that treatment groups were similar in important respects before treatments were applied?

- *Evaluating and interpreting the results*

Different questions need to be addressed depending on whether an experiment or a survey is being considered.

For an experiment:

- Is the hypothesis under test clearly stated in statistical terms?
- Does the statistical analysis appear to be appropriate?
- Is the statistical analysis presented in sufficient detail? (A P value on its own is insufficient; it should be accompanied by the numerical evidence to which it refers as well as the total numbers involved, preferably with confidence intervals.)
- Are all the people who entered the study accounted for in the analysis?
- Have statistical test procedures been interpreted correctly?
- Does the epidemiological analysis answer the research question?

For a survey:

- Have appropriate estimates been made and statistical tests performed?
- Has a multivariate analysis (if appropriate) been performed on a complete data set? How have missing observations in the data been handled?
- Have the results been correctly interpreted? Were any relevant interactions between variables overlooked?
- Does the epidemiological analysis answer the research question?

- *Final evaluation*

In weighing the evidence, the following questions might be asked:

- Was the research question worth asking in the first place, and what could be the consequences of the various possible answers? Did the research provide suggestions for action?
- Has the author made an adequate attempt to answer the question?
- Could the study design have been improved in any important way?
- Does the absence of any information from the report prevent an adequate evaluation of the study?
- Did the author take into account the results of previous studies on similar topics?

Planning a research project

Students on many basic epidemiology courses are given the task of designing a study. In some situations the exercise is taken further and the students are expected to carry out the study and analyse the data, although usually these are requirements for postgraduate students only. There is a natural progression from critical reading to the design of studies. Designing a study with adequate supervision and help from an experienced tutor is a good way of learning the principles and methods of epidemiology.

Choosing a project

The tutor should take an active role in selecting the topic and making contact with the participants in the community. Students' projects should not be too ambitious because of the inevitable shortage of time and resources. Ideally, they should be of local significance and of relevance to some health service agency, a member of which could act as a co-supervisor.

Students' projects are often group activities. Working in a group can be both beneficial and challenging, since many educational institutions encourage only individual work and achievement. Conflicts, sometimes caused by an uneven distribution of the workload, invariably have to be resolved and the involvement of a tutor at all stages is crucial to success.

The authors have had experience in two countries of organizing student projects in the fifth year of a six-year medical course. The projects involved groups of eight students in eight half-days of timetabled work. Successful projects related to topical questions that were of interest to the students. The results of the best projects have been published and many of the studies have been of great interest to health service personnel. Successful studies have dealt with:

- environmental contamination and potential health risks around a waste incinerator;
- lung cancer among iron miners;
- attitudes and behaviour in relation to the wearing of bicycle crash helmets;
- lunch-time eating habits of primary-school children;
- general practitioners' knowledge of and attitudes towards high blood cholesterol levels;
- the accuracy of ethnic classification on death certificates;
- the value of protective measures against pesticide exposure in market gardens;
- the assessment of health risks of exposure to anaesthetic gas among staff in operating theatres.

Preparation of the research protocol

The initial objective in setting out to design a study is the preparation of a written document, called a research protocol, that describes the proposed study in detail. Many points need to be addressed in a logical fashion. The following list of questions is based on that of Warren (1978).

What is the problem?

What are the general aims and the precise questions to be answered?

What will the study contribute to knowledge?
What is already known about the problem?

What study design will be used?
What are the advantages and disadvantages of this design?
Will an intervention be required?

What population will be studied?
Will a sample be necessary?
How will it be chosen?
What are the criteria for entry into the study?
How many participants are required?

What data are to be collected?
What are the variables of most interest?
What are the potential confounding variables?

How are the data to be collected?
Are the proposed methods reliable and valid?
Are appropriate quality assurance methods available?
Who will collect the data?
How will the data be recorded?
What training will the observers need?

How will the data be processed and analysed?
Is computerization necessary?
How will the data be entered?
What analyses are planned?
Who will analyse the data?
What tables and figures will be required?

Is the study ethical?
Which ethical committee will consider the protocol?
What information is required for the participants?
How will informed consent be obtained?

Will any of the participants need referral?
How will this be arranged?
What follow-up will be required?

What is the timetable for the study?
Who is responsible for each of the steps?

Is a pilot study required?
If so, how many participants are required?
How long should the pilot study last?

Will the participants in the pilot study enter the main study?

How much will the study cost?

Where will the money come from?

What resources, apart from money, are required?

How will the results of the study be publicized?

How can the results and their public health implications best be communicated to the scientific community, decision-makers and the general community?

Will a report and papers be written?

How will the participants obtain feedback?

How will the results be applied?

Conducting the project

Once the protocol has been prepared it should be circulated to a few appropriate people for comments and should subsequently be revised as necessary. With major epidemiological studies there is often a long delay between preparation of the protocol and commencement of the project, caused by the processing of a grant application. Students' projects, however, should be designed so that they can be conducted quickly and efficiently, since the time available is often very limited.

Students' projects should not require major resources, and the tutor should take responsibility for acquiring those that are necessary. The tutor should also be charged with submitting the project for ethical approval in good time.

Group projects require a reasonable division of labour and it is often helpful if a member of the group takes responsibility for liaison with the tutor. Progress should be reviewed on a regular basis and time should be allowed for the pretesting of questionnaires and for a pilot study of all aspects of the sampling and data collection process.

The project should end with a verbal presentation to the whole class (preceded, if possible, by a rehearsal) followed by a written report, which could be circulated to interested people. The report could be used for teaching purposes or as a basis for further studies.

Further reading

Over the last decade the epidemiological literature has grown enormously. Several very good textbooks for the advanced student have appeared; a list is available from Prevention of Environmental Pollution, World Health Organization, 1211 Geneva 27, Switzerland. A number of journals with a focus on epidemiology are listed in Annex 2. Mainstream medical and health journals also publish an increasing number of articles with an epidemiological content.

Various WHO publications contain useful epidemiological information. Government departments often publish material describing local epidemiological situations; for example, some departments of health statistics produce annual reports on mortality and hospital admission rates. Nongovernmental organizations such as cancer societies and heart foundations also publish material of value.

Further training

Many courses catering for people with a variety of backgrounds are now available for postgraduate training in epidemiology. WHO's regional offices, WHO agencies such as the International Agency for Research on Cancer, and nongovernmental agencies such as the International Society and Federation of Cardiology, run short courses, usually on specific topics. Short commercial summer courses are now well established in North America and Europe. Graduate courses in epidemiology, usually forming part of a master's programme in public health, are offered by universities in many parts of the world. Many of these courses have a basic broad content plus material designed for specific interests, such as cardiovascular disease epidemiology, health service evaluation, and occupational and environmental safety. A list of training courses in epidemiology is available from the Division of Environmental Health, World Health Organization, 1211 Geneva 27, Switzerland.

Study questions

11.1 The following is based on the preliminary report of a study designed to assess the value of aspirin in the prevention of coronary heart disease published in the *New England journal of medicine.*

> The Physician's Health Study is a randomized double-blind, placebo-controlled trial testing whether 325 mg of aspirin taken every other day reduces mortality from cardiovascular disease. The potentially eligible participants in the study were all male physicians 40 to 84 years of age residing in the United States at the beginning of the study in 1982. Letters of invitation, informed-consent forms, and baseline questionnaires were mailed to 261 248 such physicians identified from information on a computer tape obtained from the American Medical Association. By 31 December 1983, 112 528 had responded, of whom 59 285 were willing to participate in the trial. A large number were excluded during the enrolment phase because of poor compliance (judged by pill counts); physicians with a history of gastric bleeding and intolerance to aspirin were also excluded. 11 037 physicians were assigned at random to receive active aspirin and 11 034 to receive aspirin placebo.

This study found that aspirin had a strong protective effect against non-fatal myocardial infarction. Would you be happy to prescribe aspirin for the prevention of coronary heart disease?

11.2 The following extract is taken from a paper on asthma mortality in New Zealand, published in the *Lancet* (Wilson et al., 1981).

> *Abstract*
>
> An apparent increase in young people dying suddenly from acute asthma has been noted in the past 2 years in Auckland. 22 fatal cases were reviewed. Prescribing habits for asthma therapy have been changing in New Zealand, with a considerable increase in the use of oral theophylline drugs, particularly sustained-release preparations, which in many patients have replaced inhaled steroids and cromoglycate. It is suggested that there may be an additive toxicity between theophylline and inhaled β_2-agonists at high doses which produces cardiac arrest.
>
> *Methods*
>
> Details of deaths from asthma were obtained from the coroner's pathologist, the Auckland Asthma Society, general practitioners, and from the intensive and critical care wards of Auckland Hospital. The doctors and relatives of the patients were contacted and descriptions of mode of death and the pattern of drug administration were obtained. Statistical information on fatal asthma cases in New Zealand in the years 1974–78 was obtained from the New Zealand Department of Health. Necropsies had been performed on the 8 patients referred to the coroner.

Taking into consideration the methods used, would you agree with the suggestion that a toxic drug interaction was leading to an increased risk of death?

References

Antunes, C. M. F. et al. (1986) Controlled field trials of a vaccine against New World cutaneous leishmaniasis. *International journal of epidemiology*, **15**(4): 572–580.

Bankowski, Z. et al., ed. (1991) *Ethics and epidemiology: international guidelines. Proceedings of the XXVth CIOMS Conference.* Geneva, Council for International Organizations of Medical Sciences.

Biggar, R. J. et al. (1988) AIDS-related Kaposi's sarcoma in New York City in 1977. *New England journal of medicine*, **318**(4): 252.

Billick, I. H. et al. (1979) Analysis of pediatric blood lead levels in New York City for 1970–1976. *Environmental health perspectives*, **31**: 183–190.

Blackburn, H. (1979) Diet and mass hyperlipidemia: a public health view. In: Levy, R. et al., ed. *Nutrition, lipids and coronary heart disease.* New York, Raven Press Publishers.

Bohlin, N. I. (1967) A statistical analysis of 28 000 accident cases with emphasis on occupant restraint value. In: *SAE transactions*, Vol. 76, New York, Society of Automotive Engineers, pp. 2981–2994.

Bonita, R. & Beaglehole, R. (1989) Increased treatment of hypertension does not explain the decline in stroke mortality in the United States, 1970–1980. *Hypertension*, **13**(5) (Suppl. 1): 69–73.

Bonita, R. et al. (1990) International trends in stroke mortality, 1970–1985. *Stroke*, **21**: 989–992.

Boyes, D. A. et al. (1977) Recent results from the British Columbia screening program for cervical cancer. *American journal of obstetrics and gynecology*, **128**(6): 692–693.

Brès, P. (1986) *Public health action in emergencies caused by epidemics. A practical guide.* Geneva, World Health Organization.

Cameron, D. & Jones, I. G. (1983) John Snow, the Broad Street pump and modern epidemiology. *International journal of epidemiology*, **12**(4): 393–396.

Chigan, E. N. (1988) Integrated programme for noncommunicable disease prevention and control (NCD). *World health statistics quarterly*, **41**: 267–273.

Colditz, G. A. et al. (1988) Cigarette smoking and risk of stroke in middle-aged women. *New England journal of medicine*, **318**(15): 937–941.

Colebunders, R. et al. (1987) Evaluation of a clinical case-definition of acquired immunodeficiency syndrome in Africa. *Lancet*, **1**: 492–494.

Collins, R. et al. (1990) Blood pressure, stroke, and coronary heart disease. Part 2. Short-term reductions in blood pressure: overview of randomised drug trials in their epidemiological context. *Lancet*, **335**: 827–838.

Colton, T. (1974) *Statistics in medicine.* Boston, Little, Brown and Co.

Crane, J. et al. (1989) Prescribed fenoterol and death from asthma in New Zealand, 1981–1983: a case control study. *Lancet*, **1**: 917–922.

Crofton, J. (1987) Smoking and health in China. *Lancet*, **2**: 53.

Cummings, S. R. & Nevitt, M. C. (1989) A hypothesis: the causes of hip fracture. *Journal of gerontological medical science*, **44**: M107–111.

Curfman, G. D. (1988) Shorter hospital stay for myocardial infarction. *New England journal of medicine*, **318**(17): 1123–1125.

DARMAWAN, J. (1988) *Rheumatic conditions in the northern part of central Java: an epidemiological survey.* West Kalimantan, Geboren te Pontianak.

DIXON, W. J. & MASSEY, F. J. (1969) *Introduction to statistical analysis.* New York, McGraw Hill.

DOLL, R. & HILL, A. (1964) Mortality in relation to smoking: ten years' observations of British doctors. *British medical journal,* **1**: 1399–1410 and 1460–1467.

DRIZD, T. ET AL. (1986) *Blood pressure levels in persons 18–74 years of age in 1976–80, and trends in blood pressure from 1960 to 1980 in the United states.* Washington, DC, National Center for Health Statistics, 1986 (Vital and Health Statistics, Series 11, No. 234; DHHS publication No. (PHS) 86-1684).

EL-RAFIE, M. ET AL. (1990) Effect of diarrhoeal disease control on infant and childhood mortality in Egypt. *Lancet,* **335**: 334–338 (1990).

FARQUHAR, J. W. ET AL. (1977) Community education for cardiovascular health. *Lancet,* **1**: 1192–1195.

FENNER, F. ET AL. (1988) *Smallpox and its eradication.* Geneva, World Health Organization.

GAO, J. P. & MALISON, M. D. (1988) The epidemiology of a measles outbreak on a remote offshore island near Taiwan. *International journal of epidemiology,* **17**(4): 894–898.

GARDNER, M. J. & ALTMAN, D. G. (1986) Confidence intervals rather than P values: estimation rather than hypothesis testing. *British medical journal,* **292**(1): 746–750.

GHANA HEALTH ASSESSMENT PROJECT TEAM (1981) A quantitative method of assessing the health impact of different diseases in less developed countries. *International journal of epidemiology,* **10**(1): 73–80.

GOEDERT, J. J. ET AL. (1986) Three-year incidence of AIDS in five cohorts of HTLV-III-infected risk group members. *Science,* **231**: 992–995.

GOTTLIEB, M. S. ET AL. (1981) *Pneumocystis carinii* pneumonia and mucosal candidiasis in previously healthy homosexual men: evidence of a new acquired cellular immunodeficiency. *New England journal of medicine,* **305**(24): 1425–1431.

HAENSZEL, W. ET AL. (1972) Stomach cancer among Japanese in Hawaii. *Journal of the National Cancer Institute,* **49**(4): 969–988.

HAMMOND, E. C. ET AL. (1979) Asbestos exposure, cigarette smoking and death rates. *Annals of the New York Academy of Sciences,* **303**: 473–490.

HETZEL, B. S. (1989) *The story of iodine deficiency: an international challenge in nutrition.* New York, Oxford University Press.

HILL, A. B. (1965) The environment and disease: association or causation? *Proceedings of the Royal Society of Medicine,* **58**: 295–300.

HÖGBERG, U. & WALL, S. (1986) Secular trends in maternal mortality in Sweden from 1750 to 1980. *Bulletin of the World Health Organization,* **64**(1): 79–84.

JACKSON, R. T. & MITCHELL, E. A. (1983) Trends in hospital admission rates and drug treatment of asthma in New Zealand. *New Zealand medical journal,* **96**: 728–730.

JAMROZIK, K. ET AL. (1984) Controlled trial of three different antismoking interventions in general practice. *British medical journal,* **288**(1): 1499–1503.

KJELLSTRÖM, T. (1977) *Accumulation and renal effects of cadmium in man. A dose-response study.* Stockholm, Karolinska Institute (unpublished doctoral thesis).

KJELLSTRÖM, T. & NORDBERG, G. F. (1978) A kinetic model of cadmium metabolism in the human being. *Environmental research,* **16**(1–3): 248–269.

KJELLSTRÖM, T. ET AL. (1982) Comparison of mercury in hair with fish-eating habits of children in Auckland. *Community health studies,* **6**: 57–63.

LAST, J. M. (1988) *A dictionary of epidemiology*. 2nd ed. Oxford, Oxford University Press.

LAST, J. M. (1990) *Guidelines on ethics for epidemiologists*. International Epidemiological Association, 1990 (unpublished discussion document).

LIPID RESEARCH CLINICS PROGRAM (1984) The lipid research clinics coronary primary prevention trial results. 1. Reduction in incidence of coronary heart disease. *Journal of the American Medical Association*, **251**(3): 351–364.

LU, J.-B. & QIN, Y.-M. (1987) Correlation between high salt intake and mortality rates for oesophageal and gastric cancers in Henan Province, China. *International journal of epidemiology*, **16**(2): 171–176.

LUCAS, D. & KANE, P., ed. (1985) *Asking demographic questions*. Canberra, National Centre for Development Studies, Australian National University (Demography Teaching Notes, Series No. 5).

LWANGA, S. K. & LEMESHOW, S. (1991) *Sample size determination in health studies*. Geneva, World Health Organization.

LWANGA, S. K. & TYE, C.-Y. (1986) *Teaching health statistics: twenty lesson and seminar outlines*. Geneva, World Health Organization.

McDONALD, J. C. ET AL. (1980) Chrysolite fibre concentration and lung cancer mortality: a preliminary report. In: Wagner, J. C., ed. *Biological effects of mineral fibres*. Vol. 2. Lyons, International Agency for Research on Cancer (IARC Scientific Publications, No. 30), pp. 811–817.

McGINNIS, J. M. (1990) Settting objectives for public health in the 1990s: experience and prospects. *Annual review of public health*, **11**: 231–249.

McKEOWN, T. (1976) *The role of medicine: dream, mirage or nemesis*? London, Nuffield Provincial Hospitals Trust.

McKINLAY, J. B. ET AL. (1989) A review of the evidence concerning the impact of medical measures on recent mortality and morbidity in the United States. *International journal of health services*, **19**(2): 181–208.

McMICHAEL, A. J. (1976) Standardized mortality ratios and the "healthy worker effect": scratching beneath the surface. *Journal of occupational medicine*, **18**(3): 165–168.

McMICHAEL, A. J. (1991) Macro-environmental problems and health: the penny drops at last. *Medical journal of Australia*, **154**: 499–501.

MANTON, K. G. (1988) The global impact of noncommunicable diseases: estimation and projection. *World health statistics quarterly*, **41**(3/4): 255–266.

MASIRONI, R. & ROTHWELL, C. (1988) Tendances et effets du tabagisme dans le monde [Smoking trends and effects worldwide]. *World health statistics quarterly*, **41**(3/4): 228–241 (in French, with English summary).

MEDICAL RESEARCH COUNCIL WORKING PARTY (1985) MRC trial of treatment of mild hypertension: prinicipal results. *British medical journal*, **291**(2): 97–104.

MELLIN, G. W. & KATZENSTEIN, M. (1962) The saga of thalidomide: neuropathy to embryopathy, with case reports of congenital anomalies. *New England journal of medicine*, **267**(23): 1184–1193; **267**(24): 1238–1244.

MILLS, A. (1985) Survey and examples of economic evaluation of health programmes in developing countries. *World health statistics quarterly*, **38**(4): 402–31.

MILLAR, J. S. ET AL. (1985) Meat consumption as a risk factor in enteritis necroticans. *International journal of epidemiology*, **14**(2): 318–321.

MILLER, A. B. ET AL. (1976) Mortality from cancer of the uterus in Canada and its relationship to screening for cancer of the cervix. *International journal of cancer*, **17**: 602–612.

MOLLA, A. M. ET AL. (1985) Rice-based oral rehydration solution decreases the stool volume in acute diarrhoea. *Bulletin of the World Health Organization*, **63**(4): 751–756.

MUSHAK, P. ET AL. (1989) Prenatal and postnatal effects of low-level lead exposure: integrated summary of a report of the US Congress on childhood lead poisoning. *Environmental research*, **50**(1): 11–36.

NEEDLEMAN, H. L. ET AL. (1979) Deficits in psychologic and classroom performance of children with elevated dentine lead levels. *New England journal of medicine*, **300**(13): 689–695.

NEW ZEALAND DEPARTMENT OF HEALTH (1989) *New Zealand health goals and targets*. Wellington.

OTTAWA CHARTER for HEALTH PROMOTION (1986) *Health promotion*, **1**(4): i–v.

PEARCE, N. & JACKSON, R. (1988) Statistical testing and estimation in medical research. *New Zealand medical journal*, **101**: 569–570.

PRINEAS, R. J. ET AL. (1982) *The Minnesota code manual of electrocardiographic findings: standards and procedures for measurement and classification*. Stoneham, MA, Butterworth Publications.

ROBINE, J.-M. (1989) Estimation de la valeur de l'espérance de vie sans incapacité (EVSI) pour les pays occidentaux au cours de la dernière décennie: quelle peut-être l'utilité de ce nouvel indicateur de l'état de santé? [Estimating disability-free life expectancy (DFLE) in the Western countries in the last decade: how can this new indicator of health status be used?] *World health statistics quarterly*, **42**(3): 141–150 (in French, with English summary).

ROSE, G. (1985) Sick individuals and sick populations. *International journal of epidemiology*, **14**(1): 32–38.

ROSS, D. A. & VAUGHAN, J. D. (1986) Health interview surveys in developing countries: a methodological review. *Studies in family planning*, **17**: 78–94.

SACKETT, D. L. ET AL. (1985) *Clinical epidemiology: a basic science for clinical medicine*. Boston, Little, Brown and Co.

SACKS, H. S. ET AL. (1987) Meta-analysis of randomised controlled trials. *New England journal of medicine*, **316**: 450–455.

SAID, S. ET AL. (1985) Seroepidemiology of hepatitis B in a population of children in central Tunisia. *International journal of epidemiology*, **14**(2): 313–317.

SALONEN, J. T. ET AL. (1986) Analysis of community-based cardiovascular disease prevention studies: evaluation issues in the North Karelia Project and the Minnesota Heart Health Program. *International journal of epidemiology*, **15**(2): 176–182 (1986).

SCHILTS, R. (1988) *And the band played on*. New York, Penguin Books.

SHAPIRO, S. (1989) Determining the efficacy of breast cancer screening. *Cancer*, **63**(10): 1873–1880.

SIEGEL, S. & CASTERLLAN (1988) *Nonparametric statistics for the behavioural sciences*, 2nd ed. New York, McGraw Hill.

SMITH, G. S. (1989) Development of rapid epidemiologic assessment methods to evaluate health status and delivery of health services. *International journal of epidemiology*, **18**(4) (Suppl. 2): 2–15.

SNOW, J. (1855) *On the mode of communication of cholera*. London, Churchill (Reprinted in *Snow on cholera: a reprint of two papers*. New York, Hafner Publishing Company, 1965).

STEERING COMMITTEE OF THE PHYSICIANS' HEALTH STUDY RESEARCH GROUP (1988) Preliminary report: findings from the aspirin component of the ongoing physicians' health study. *New England journal of medicine*, **318**(4): 262–264.

STEWART, A. W. ET AL. (1984) Trends in survival after myocardial infarction in New Zealand, 1974–1981. *Lancet*, **2**: 444–446.

SYME, L. & GURALNIK, J. M. (1987) Epidemiology and health policy: coronary heart disease. In: Levine, S. & Lilienfeld, A. M., ed. *Epidemiology and health policy*. New York, Tavistock Publications (Contemporary Issues in Health, Medicine and Social Policy), pp. 85–116.

TARANTA, A. & MARKOWITZ, M. (1989) *Rheumatic fever: a guide to its recognition, prevention and cure*, 2nd ed. Lancaster, Kluwer Academic Publishers.

TOPOL, E. J. ET AL. (1988) A randomized controlled trial of hospital discharge three days after myocardial infarction in the era of reperfusion. *New England journal of medicine*, **318**(17): 1083–1088.

TUGWELL, P. ET AL. (1985) The measurement iterative loop: a framework for the critical appraisal of need, benefits and costs of health interventions. *Journal of chronic diseases*, **38**(4): 339–351.

TUOMILEHTO, J. ET AL. (1986) Smoking rates in Pacific islands. *Bulletin of the World Health Organization*, **64**(3): 447–456.

UEMURA, K. & PISA, Z. (1988) Trends in cardiovascular disease mortality in industralized countries since 1950. *World health statistics quarterly*, **41**(3/4): 155–178.

UNITED KINGDOM GOVERNMENT STATISTICAL SERVICE (1984) *Press notice on seat belt use in Great Britain*. London, Department of Transport.

UNITED KINGDOM MINISTRY OF HEALTH (1954) *Mortality and morbidity during the London fog of December* 1952. London, Her Majesty's Stationery Office.

UNICEF (1987) *The state of the world's children 1987*. New York, Oxford University Press.

UNITED NATIONS (1984) *Handbook of household surveys*, revised edition. New York (Studies in Methods, Series F, No. 31).

UNITED STATES PUBLIC HEALTH SERVICE (1964) *Smoking and health: report of the advisory committee to the Surgeon General of the Public Health Service*. Washington, DC (PHS Publication No. 1103).

UNITED STATES DEPARTMENT OF HEALTH AND HUMAN SERVICES (1986) *The 1990 health objectives for the nation: a mid-course review*. Washington, DC.

VAUGHAN, J. P. & MORROW, R. H. (1989) *Manual of epidemiology for district health management*. Geneva, World Health Organization.

VICTORA, C. G. ET AL. (1987) Birthweight and infant mortality: a longitudinal study of 5,914 Brazilian children. *International journal of epidemiology*, **16**(2): 239–245.

WARREN, M. D. (1978) Aide-mémoire for preparing a protocol. *British medical journal*, **1**: 1195–1196.

WILLIAMS, A. (1985) Economics of coronary artery bypass grafting. *British medical journal*, **291**: 326–329.

WILSON, J. D. ET AL. (1981) Has the change to beta-agonists combined with oral theophylline increased cases of fatal asthma? *Lancet*, **1**: 1235–1237.

WILSON, J. M. G. & JÜNGNER, G. (1968) *Principles and practice of screening for disease*. Geneva, World Health Organization (Public Health Papers, No. 34).

WHO (1976) *Mercury*. Geneva, World Health Organization (Environmental Health Criteria, No. 1).

WHO (1977) *Lead*. Geneva, World Health Organization (Environmental Health Criteria, No. 3).

WHO (1980a) *Noise*. Geneva, World Health Organization (Environmental Health Criteria, No. 12).

WHO (1980b) *International classification of impairments, disabilities and handicaps. A manual of classification relating to the consequences of disease*. Geneva, World Health Organization.

WHO (1980c) *Recommended health-based limits in occupational exposure to heavy metals: report of a WHO Study Group*. Geneva, World Health Organization (WHO Technical Report Series, No. 647).

WHO (1982) *Prevention of coronary heart disease: report of a WHO Expert Committee.* Geneva, World Health Organization (WHO Technical Report Series, No. 678).

WHO (1985) *Diabetes mellitus: report of a WHO Study Group.* Geneva, World Health Organization (WHO Technical Report Series, No. 727).

WHO (1986) Acquired immunodeficiency syndrome (AIDS). WHO/CDC case definition for AIDS. *Weekly epidemiological record,* **61**(10), 69–76.

WHO (1987a) *World health statistics annual 1986.* Geneva, World Health Organization.

WHO (1987b) WHO report. *AIDS action,* **1**: 1–5

WHO (1987c) *Early detection of occupational diseases.* Geneva, World Health Organization.

WHO (1987d) *Air quality guidelines for Europe.* Copenhagen, WHO Regional Office for Europe (Regional Publications, European Series, No. 23).

WHO (1988a) *Rheumatic fever and rheumatic heart disease: report of a WHO Study Group.* Geneva, World Health Organization (WHO Technical Report Series, No. 764).

WHO (1988b) *Derived intervention levels for radionuclides in food. Guidelines for application after widespread radioactive contamination.* Geneva, World Health Organization.

WHO (1989a) *Report of the first meeting of the technical advisory group.* Geneva, 6–10 March 1989. Unpublished document No. WHO/ARI/89.4; available on request from Division of Diarrhoeal and Acute Respiratory Disease Control, World Health Organization, 1211 Geneva 27, Switzerland.

WHO (1989b) *Weekly epidemiological record,* **64**(2): 5–12.

WHO (1989c) *Assessment and management of environmental health hazards.* Unpublished document No. WHO/PEP/89.6; available on request from Division of Environmental Health, World Health Organization, 1211 Geneva 27, Switzerland.

WHO (1990a) *World health statistics annual 1989.* Geneva, World Health Organization.

WHO (1990b) *Methylmercury.* Geneva, World Health Organization (Environmental Health Criteria, No. 101).

WHO (1992a) *Weekly epidemiological record,* **67**: 97–98.

WHO (1992b) *International statistical classification of diseases and related health problems. Tenth revision.* Vol. 1. Geneva, World Health Organization.

WHO (1993) *Management of acute respiratory infections in children. Practical guidelines for outpatient care.* Geneva, World Health Organization, in press.

WHO/UNEP (1988) *GEMS assessment of urban air quality.* Geneva, World Health Organization (unpublished WHO document No. PEP/88.2; available on request from Division of Environmental Health, World Health Organization, 1211 Geneva 27, Switzerland).

YUSUF, S. ET AL. (1985) Beta blockade during and after myocardial infarction: an overview of the randomized trials. *Progress in cardiovascular diseases,* **27**(5): 335–371.

Annex 1

Answers to study questions

1.1 The fact that there were over 40 times more cholera cases in one district than in the other does not reflect the risk of catching cholera in the two districts. It is not appropriate to compare the number of deaths in the two groups since the population supplied by the Southwark Company was over eight times larger than the population supplied by the Lambeth Company. Death rates (number of deaths divided by the population supplied) must be compared. In fact the death rate in the population supplied by the Southwark Company was over five times greater than that in the Lambeth district.

1.2 The best evidence would come from intervention studies. The 1854 epidemic was controlled in a most dramatic manner when the handle of a water pump was removed. The epidemic died away rapidly, although the evidence suggests (and Snow knew) that the epidemic was already waning before this act. More convincing was the reduction in cholera rates in the population supplied by the Lambeth Company in the period 1849–54 (before the epidemic) after the Company had begun extracting water from a less contaminated part of the River Thames.

1.3 Doctors make a good study group because they comprise a well-defined occupational group with similar socioeconomic status, and are relatively easy to follow up. They are also likely to be interested in health matters and cooperative in this type of study.

1.4 It can be concluded that lung cancer death rates increase dramatically with the number of cigarettes smoked. From the data alone it is not possible to conclude that smoking causes lung cancer; some other factor associated with smoking might be causing the disease. However, in 1964, on the basis of this study and many others, the United States Surgeon General concluded that lung cancer was caused by cigarette smoking.

1.5 The distribution of the population is the first factor to consider. The concentration of cases in one area is interesting only if the population is spread throughout that area. Secondly, it needs to be known whether the search for cases has been as intensive in the areas without cases as in the area with cases. During the Minamata disease outbreak, an intensive search was made throughout the whole region and it was found that several large population centres had no cases.

1.6 The reported occurrence of rheumatic fever has declined dramatically in Denmark since the early 1900s. It could be a real decline although it would be important to try to rule out the influence of changes in diagnostic fashion and reporting practices. Since effective medical treatment for rheumatic fever became available only in the 1940s, most of the decline has been due to socioeconomic improvements, e.g. in housing and nutrition. It is also possible that the responsible organism has become less virulent.

1.7 Men who do not smoke and are not exposed to asbestos dust have the lowest lung cancer rates, followed in increasing order by men exposed to asbestos dust alone, men who smoke but are not exposed to asbestos dust, and finally men who both smoke and are exposed to asbestos dust. This is an example of interaction in which two factors work together to produce a very high rate of disease. From a public health perspective it is important to ensure that people exposed to asbestos dust do not smoke, and, of course, to reduce exposure to the dust.

2.1 The three measures are prevalence rate, incidence rate and cumulative incidence. Prevalence rate is the proportion of the population affected by a disease or condition at a given point in time and is approximately equal to the incidence rate multiplied by the duration of disease. Incidence rate measures the rate at which new events occur in a population; it can take into account variable time periods during which individuals are disease-free. Cumulative incidence measures the denominator (i.e. the population at risk) at only one point in time (usually at the beginning of a study) and thus measures the risk of individuals contracting a disease during a specified period.

2.2 Prevalence rate is a useful measure of the frequency of non-insulin-dependent diabetes because diabetes has a relatively low incidence and because a very large population and a long study period would be required in order to find sufficient new cases to measure incidence rate. The variation shown in Table 2.2 could reflect differences in measurement. The adequacy of the methods used in the various surveys would need to be assessed; survey response rates and laboratory methods would have to be looked at, among other things. It should be noted, however, that standard criteria are being applied on the basis of blood glucose levels after a standard glucose load. It is likely that much of the variation in diabetes prevalence is real and due, at least in part, to variations in diet, exercise and other elements of lifestyle.

2.3 Age standardization ensures that differences in death rates are not due simply to differences in age distribution in the populations. The first possible explanation for the variation between groups relates to the quality of the information on the death certificate. It is necessary to establish that differences are real and not due to varying diagnostic or certification practices. In fact the differences have been shown to be real. The variation in death rates may be due to variation in either incidence rates or case–fatality.

2.4 Risk difference and risk ratio (see pages 28–30).

2.5 Although the relative risk is only about 1.5 the population attributable risk is about 20% (i.e. about 20% of the cases of lung cancer in a typical population of a developed country can be attributed to passive smoking). This is because up to half the population is exposed to passive smoking.

3.1 The main epidemiological study designs are the cross-sectional survey, the case–control study, the cohort study and the randomized control trial. Their relative strengths and weaknesses are summarized in the text and in Tables 3.5 and 3.6.

3.2 The case–control study would start with cases of bowel cancer, preferably newly diagnosed ones, and a group of controls (without the disease) from the same source population (to avoid selection bias). The cases and controls would be asked about their usual diet in the past. Measurement bias could be a problem. It is difficult to remember past diet with great accuracy, and the development of the disease might influence recall. The analysis would compare the content of the diet in the cases and controls, controlling for possible confounding variables.

In a cohort study, detailed data on diet are collected in a large group of people free of bowel disease; the cohort is followed up for several years and all new cases of bowel cancer are identified. The risk of disease is then related to the fat content of the diet at the beginning and during the study. This study design presents many logistic problems but systematic bias is less of a problem.

3.3 Random error is the variation of an observed value from the true population value due to chance alone. It can be reduced by increasing the size of the study sample and improving the reliability of the measurement method.

3.4 Systematic error occurs when there is a tendency to produce results that differ systematically from the true values. The main sources of systematic error are selection bias and measurement bias.

Selection bias occurs when the people who take part in a study are systematically different from those who do not. The possibility of selection bias can be reduced by a clear and explicit definition of the criteria for entry into the study, a knowledge of the natural history and management of the disease, and a high response rate.

Measurement bias occurs when there is a systematic error in measurement or classification of the participants in a study, It can be reduced by good study design, involving, for example, standard criteria for the disease, detailed attention to the quality control of measurement methods, and the collection of data without knowledge of the disease status of the participant.

4.1 The approximate estimates of the arithmetic mean and the median are 1 and 0.75 respectively. The values differ because the distribution is skewed.

4.2 There is no right or wrong answer to this question. A one-tailed test can be justified if the researcher has evidence that the probability of low doses of medication having greater therapeutic value than high doses is negligible. It is also justified if the researcher is only interested in testing the one-sided hypothesis. On the other hand, if therapeutic effects may decline with increased doses the two-tailed test is necessary.

4.3 In examining a variable with a highly skewed distribution, such as per capita income, the median would be a more useful measure of central tendency than the mean.

5.1 The process of determining whether an observed association is likely to be causal.

5.2 This statement is reasonable because, ultimately, evidence from human populations (epidemiological evidence) is usually required before a conclusion can be drawn on the causal nature of an association. However, many other scientific disciplines contribute to causal inference.

5.3 The criteria include: the temporal nature of the relation, plausibility, consistency, the strength of the association, the dose–response relationship, reversibility, and the study design. Of these criteria, only temporality is essential; ultimately, judgement is required.

5.4 On the basis of this evidence alone one could not be certain that the association was causal; a policy of withdrawing the drug could not, therefore, be recommended. The effects of bias (measurement, selection) and confounding in the study and the role of chance would need to be assessed. If bias and chance are unlikely to be the explanation, then the causal criteria can be applied. In fact, when all the evidence was considered in such a study in New Zealand, the investigators concluded that the association was likely to be causal (Crane et al., 1989).

5.5 A temporal relationship is most important. Did the patients consume the oil before or after they fell ill? If there is no information on the chemical in the oil that is associated with the disease, it is impossible to assess plausibility or consistency. Therefore strength and dose–response relationship based on information on oil consumption could be the next matters for study. As it is urgent to find the likely cause, the most suitable approach would be to conduct a case–control study, together with chemical analysis of the oil and of biological monitoring samples. If would be prudent to intervene as soon as a temporal relationship has been clearly established and the strength of association appears great, particularly if there is no other likely cause.

6.1 The four levels of prevention are: primordial, primary, secondary and tertiary. A comprehensive programme for the prevention of tuberculosis would include activities at each of these levels.

Primordial prevention would involve stopping the entry of the tubercle bacillus into the community. People from endemic areas can be required to provide evidence that they are not infected before entering non-endemic areas. In addition, the factors that increase the risk of tuberculosis, such as overcrowding, poverty and poor nutrition can be dealt with.

Primary prevention includes immunization and case-finding, to avoid spread of the disease.

Secondary prevention programmes would involve the early and effective treatment of infected people.

Tertiary prevention involves rehabilitation of patients suffering from the long-term effects or sequelae of tuberculosis and its treatment.

6.2 For a disease to be suitable for screening it must be serious, the natural history of the disease must be understood, there should be a long period between development of the first signs and appearance of overt disease, an effective treatment must be available and, usually, the prevalence of the disease must be high.

6.3 All study designs have been used to evaluate screening programmes. Randomized controlled trials are ideal, but cross-sectional, cohort and case–control studies are also used.

7.1 The proportion of deaths due to infectious diseases has declined in the USA since 1950 and chronic diseases have become more important. Demographic change, with an increased proportion of elderly people, is one explanation. It would be helpful to have age-specific mortality data for individual diseases to allow further examination of the trends. Two general explanations for a decrease in age-specific infectious disease mortality have been advanced. First, there has been a general reduction in host susceptibility through improved nutrition and sanitation. This is likely to be the most important factor, particularly in respect of the early improvement. Secondly, specific medical interventions may have played a part, particularly since the 1950s.

7.2 A record of weekly (or daily) cases of measles found by clinics and health practitioners in the district should be kept. The "normal" background level (perhaps two cases or fewer per week) and a threshold level for an incipient epidemic (perhaps twice or three times the background level) should be established. When the threshold is exceeded, preventive action should be taken. For further details, see Vaughan & Morrow (1989).

7.3 The chain of infection for foodborne salmonella goes from faecal material (either from human beings or animals, particularly chickens) to water or food which, when consumed, leads to infection. Alternatively, it goes from faecal material to hands and then to food (during food preparation), which again leads to infection.

8.1 The term is strictly a contradiction in that epidemiology deals with populations whereas clinical medicine deals with individual patients. However, it is appropriate because clinical epidemiology studies populations of patients.

8.2 The limitation of this definition is that there are no biological grounds for using an arbitrary cut-off point as the basis for distinguishing normal from abnormal. For many diseases the risk increases with increasing levels of risk factors and much of the burden of disease falls on people in the normal range.

8.3 The sensitivity of the new test $= 8/10 \times 100 = 80\%$; its specificity $= 9000/10\,000 \times 100 = 90\%$. The new test appears good; a decision on whether to use it in the general population requires information on its positive predictive value, which in this case is $8/1008 = 0.008$. This very low value is related to the low prevalence of the disease. For this reason, it would not be appropriate to recommend general use of the test.

8.4 The positive predictive value of a screening test is the proportion of the people with positive results who actually have the disease. The major determinant of the positive predictive value is the prevalence of the preclinical disease in the screened population. If the population is at low risk for the disease, most of the positive results will be false. Predictive value also depends on the sensitivity and specificity of the test.

9.1 (a) For FEP in red blood cells, and probably also for ALAD.
(b) Children.

9.2 (a) An increasing relative risk of lung cancer.

(b) Because it is known that the total amount (dose) of asbestos particles (fibres) inhaled (concentration × duration of exposure) is what determines the risk of asbestos-induced disease.

9.3 (a) The worker group needs to be stratified according to duration of exposure. Those with less than three months' exposure will have lower blood levels than the other workers, even though they have experienced the same exposure situation.

(b) A new cadmium exposure situation would be characterized by high average blood cadmium in the population while urine cadmium is still low. A problem of many years' standing would lead to high cadmium levels in both blood and urine.

9.4 You should start by collecting case histories, holding discussions with local medical services and making visits to suspected industries in order to develop the hypothesis for study. Then a case–control study of lung cancer within the city should be carried out.

9.5 Information on deaths in previous years (without smog) and on the age-specific causes of death would be helpful. Evidence from animal experiments might serve to document the effects of the smog (in fact, animals on display at London's Smithfield Meat Market also suffered). The close time association of the smog and its pollutants with an increase in deaths is strong evidence for a causal relationship.

9.6 The healthy worker effect refers to the low background morbidity and mortality rates that are found in both exposed and unexposed groups in the workplace. The reason is that, in order to be active in an occupation, people need to be reasonably healthy. Ill and disabled people are selectively excluded from the study groups. If a control group is chosen from the general population, bias may be introduced because the group is inherently less healthy.

10.1 Various questions must be asked at different stages of the planning cycle:

How common are falls in the elderly?

What epidemiological data are available?

What studies are required?

How can falls be prevented?

What treatment resources are available?

How effective are the treatment services?

What rehabilitation services are available and are they effective?

How does the cost of these services compare with their effectiveness?

Should new types of services be established and tested?

Has the occurrence of falls changed since the new services were provided?

10.2 The health promotion strategies involve building healthy public policy, creating supportive environments, strengthening community action, developing personal skills, and reorienting health services.

With regard to cigarette smoking, a healthy public policy would involve action by the agricultural sector to encourage crops other than tobacco, fiscal measures to increase the tax on tobacco, and trade decisions to restrict its importation. A supportive environment would be aided by a ban on the advertising and promotion of tobacco products. Community action would be strengthened by the encouragement of no-smoking areas in public places. Educating smokers in techniques to stop smoking would be helpful. The health services could encourage smoking control measures, such as restrictions on smoking in all public facilities and help for high-risk smokers, among them pregnant women and patients with cardiovascular and respiratory diseases.

11.1 This was a well-designed and well-conducted randomized controlled trial on the use of aspirin in the primary prevention of cardiovascular mortality. The study was conducted on male American physicians who, it turned out, were very healthy. Out of a total of 261 000 physicians, 22 000 took part. The healthy state of the physicians meant that the study had less statistical power than originally planned. Extrapolating the results to other populations is difficult because of the exclusions that limited the study population to physicians likely to comply and not to have adverse side-effects. These design features increased the likelihood of a high success rate. Confirmation of the benefits of aspirin is required from other studies. It is always necessary to balance benefits against risks (gastrointestinal side-effects, increased risk of bleeding, etc.).

11.2 Ecological evidence on asthma therapy is related to a suggested increase in asthma mortality. It would be difficult to agree with the conclusion. Information is presented only on people dying with asthma; no information is provided on asthmatics not dying. This study is a case series; there are no controls. Such a study, however, points to the desirability of further investigation. In this case a more formal examination of asthma mortality trends has identified a new epidemic of asthma deaths, the cause of which is still under investigation, although a particular drug has apparently contributed substantially to it.

Annex 2
Epidemiology journals

American journal of epidemiology

The official journal of the Society for Epidemiologic Research, published twice monthly. It contains a wide range of reviews, commentaries and original papers in all branches of epidemiology, with an emphasis on etiological research.
Further information from: American journal of epidemiology, 2007E Monument Street, Baltimore, MD 21205, USA.

Annals of epidemiology

The official journal of the American College of Epidemiology. Produced quarterly, it publishes reports of original research on the epidemiology of chronic and acute diseases for clinicians and public health researchers.
Further information from: Annals of epidemiology, Brigham and Women's Hospital, Harvard Medical School, 55 Pond Avenue, Brookline, MA 02146, USA.

Bulletin of the World Health Organization

This bimonthly journal publishes original articles in English or French, with a summary in the other language, by authors from all areas of the world.
Further information from: Editor, Bulletin of the World Health Organization, World Health Organization, 1211 Geneva 27, Switzerland.

Epidemiologic reviews

This annual journal is sponsored by the Society for Epidemiologic Research and the International Epidemiology Association. It publishes major review articles on key issues in epidemiology and public health.
Further information from: American journal of epidemiology, 2007 E Monument Street, Baltimore, MD 21205, USA.

Epidemiology

Published bimonthly by Williams and Wilkins and Epidemiology Resources Inc., this journal deals with all aspects of epidemiology.
Further information from: Epidemiology, Williams and Wilkins, 248 E Preston Street, Baltimore, MD 21202, USA.

European journal of epidemiology

This bimonthly journal publishes articles on the epidemiology of communicable and noncommunicable diseases and their control.
Further information from: European journal of epidemiology, Via Zandona 11, 00194 Rome, Italy.

International journal of epidemiology

The official journal of the International Epidemiological Association. Produced monthly, it publishes original work, reviews and letters to the editor on research and teaching in epidemiology. All papers are available in English although the submission of articles in other languages is acceptable. Each issue contains numerous articles covering a wide range of topics.
Further information from: Journal Subscriptions Department, Oxford University Press, Walton Street, Oxford OX2 60P, England.

Journal of clinical epidemiology

Formerly the *Journal of chronic diseases*, this journal is published monthly. It is concerned with research on chronic illness and clinical epidemiology. Articles are published on methods as well as on the results of research.
Further information from: Journal of clinical epidemiology, Yale University School of Medicine, 333 Cedar Street, P.O. Box 3333, New Haven, CT 06510-8025, USA.

Journal of epidemiology and community health

Published quarterly by the British Medical Association, this journal carries original work in the fields of epidemiology, community health and the organization and functioning of health services.
Further information from: British medical journal, BMA House, Tavistock Square, London WC1H 9JR, England.

Revue d'épidémiologie et de santé publique [Epidemiology and public health]

Published quarterly. Articles in French and English covering original work in epidemiology, community health and assessment of health services.
Further information from: INSERM, U 149, 123 Boulevard de Port-Royal, F-75014 Paris, France.

World health statistics quarterly

This quarterly journal publishes articles in English or French, with a summary in the other language. Each issue has a theme and articles are generally invited by WHO, but submitted original articles will also be considered.
Further information from: Editor, World health statistics quarterly, World Health Organization, 1211 Geneva 27, Switzerland.

Index